Reinvent the Heal

A Philosophy for The Reform of Medical Practice

James T. Hansen, M.D.

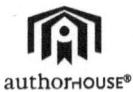
authorHOUSE®

AuthorHouse™
1663 Liberty Drive
Bloomington, IN 47403
www.authorhouse.com
Phone: 1-800-839-8640

© 2012 James T. Hansen, M.D. All rights reserved.

No part of this book may be reproduced, stored in a retrieval system, or transmitted by any means without the written permission of the author.

Published by AuthorHouse 7/9/2012

ISBN : 978-1-4772-1148-9 (sc)
ISBN: 978-1-4772-1147-2 (dj)
ISBN: 978-1-4772-1146-5 (e)

Library of Congress Control Number: 2012909696

Any people depicted in stock imagery provided by Thinkstock are models, and such images are being used for illustrative purposes only.
Certain stock imagery © Thinkstock.

This book is printed on acid-free paper.

Because of the dynamic nature of the Internet, any web addresses or links contained in this book may have changed since publication and may no longer be valid. The views expressed in this work are solely those of the author and do not necessarily reflect the views of the publisher, and the publisher hereby disclaims any responsibility for them.

Prologue

We have all witnessed health care in America being transformed into a complex tangle of economical, technological and ethical issues. As the cauldron continues to boil, voices clamor from every side. Physicians fight insurance companies for control and profits, consumers hold out for the latest treatments and cures, hospitals flounder over which side of the battlefield to choose. It's a witches' brew, stirred by money, greed and control, with the real mission of medicine pushed to the sidelines while power attempts to wrest control of the industry.

Yet this complex tangle has as its foundation the physician-patient encounter. This is the point from which all other activities flow – the spark that ignites the rest of the industry. This is ground zero, hallowed ground where a moment is born, one that fuses the strengths of healer and patient, where a covenant springs forth promising the restoration of health. Decisions to add hospital beds, build new clinics, medical schools and specialty wings, purchase MRI machines, form an HMO or develop a state-of-the-art trauma center are all born from this very important point of service, yet these secondary considerations often eclipse the process of healing and not infrequently lead to an adulteration of the symbiosis between doctor and patient. It is tempting to place blame for the healthcare crisis at the feet of the government, insurance companies, pharmaceutical companies, attorneys, legislators, hospitals or health care engineers, but the target is clearly where physicians and patients interact. While it is the physician who ultimately makes the decision as to what must be done, it is we patients who have stood by, handing over trust where it has not been earned, silently acquiescing while our doctors make outrageous decisions, ultimately jacking up the cost of healthcare. This is the lowest common denominator, the irreducible process, the core from which springs the success or failure of the enterprise. If there are problems in the industry, then this is the place to look for root causes. As both a physician and a patient I have come to believe that physician and patient responsibility are unavoidable and we patients need to clearly understand that without substantial change poor heath care will clearly be the winner. So poor health care or mediocrity is one of the certain casualties of an unhealthy physician-patient relationship. But there is more.

Why have the costs of health care grown at such an alarming rate? There is a clear cut parallel between the rise of mediocrity and health care expenditures. At first glance it would appear that as medical technology evolves, as it becomes more sophisticated, then our individual and corporate health should improve. That is not what is happening. How do well intentioned and well-trained physicians play such a major role in driving up these costs? What becomes of their altruism when they graduate from medical school?. How have they managed to drive up costs and maintain their stature at the same time? How is it possible to have the most technologically sophisticated health care system in the world and still see so much suffering, especially with chronic diseases? Chronic diseases now account for nearly one third of the health care burden. They account for much of the health care dollar and we have learned that they do not respond to the standard allopathic approach.

By the same token, how can we patients be so acquiescent, so passive, and so trusting of the process. How is it that we are so insensitive to the real costs and the potential complication of the excesses of high tech medicine?

I am here to tell you that the system is falling apart. I have been in this doctoring business for 40 years and I have witnessed the disintegration of those strengths, which foster healing, which lead to bountiful life, and which facilitate the transfer of meaningful medical advancement to patients. The decay of this system is closely tied to the excesses of technomedicine, the overuse of high technology in the practice of medicine, and something positive needs to happen or mediocrity will triumph. Health care is a mandate for all citizens, but the operative phrase is quality health care. This current debacle did not occur by happenstance. Consider the excesses in health care decisions made by physicians in the last few decades of this century. Extravagance was the model we older physicians left for new physicians and their patients. At the same time, we patients were asleep at the switch, as if high technology could solve all of our health care needs and provide us with immortality. Some legacy! And, indeed, the buck stops at the doctor-patient interface. It is the "physician's pen"—i.e., the decisions he or she makes—that generates the cascade of events that follow from this sacrosanct encounter. We patients have not played an active part in the activation of the physicians pen. Ignorance is not an excuse. The power of the physician's pen has been astonishing and is only now being challenged. This is one locus where reform can occur.

But how did this all happen? And -- by relieving physicians of autonomy, power, discretion and authority, do we lose something in our new health care reality? Is there enough incentive to keep dedicated individuals committed to the rigorous training and long hours? Will physicians be replaced by health care teams? What went wrong?

I have attempted to answer these questions. This is one person's point of view, but it has been infused and nourished by nearly two generations of practicing medicine, teaching, physician leadership, and my own emotional evolution. The book is divided into four parts:

1. Backdrop: The problem is spelled out. Its genesis is outlined. These first two chapters are a call to arms. The facts are laid bare. Ground zero is defined.
2. Chapters 3-14 provide the reader with the journey. Much as Dante described his descent into Hell, this is where the health care debacle is described, where the undersurface of medical practice is explored. It is through this journey that my own awareness was given expression.
3. The last three chapters culminate with a vision. We ascend from the depths of dysfunction to a way out. This will only work when we citizens understand that only by taking action can this dysfunction be repaired. The case is made for a national dialogue. The kinds of action we citizens can take are dealt with in the last chapter

Chapter 1
A Portrait Of Catastrophe: Where We Are And How We Got Here

At times meaning simply precipitates out of nothingness and puts a lasting border around the moment. The bus was heading in the opposite direction but anyone could see the malevolent invitation that it conveyed. The brightly colored advertisement clung tenaciously to the side of the bus, carefully conveying a message designed to hit its mark, boldly announcing a new medical test, which would both ensure health and detect illness early in its course. But, a body CT scan? A *body* CT scan, is a very sophisticated version of snake oil. CT scans have been a very important advancement in the specialty of radiology. They have allowed physicians to use x-rays and penetrate the various layers of tissue to more carefully define an abnormality suspected. Most CT radiography is applied to a specific area, an area of the body identified by other less invasive tests likely to yield additional information regarding a suspected malady. But a body CT scan represents a shotgun approach, more likely to identify innocent variations that are normal and simply part of the individuality so characteristic of human beings. So here was this bus, of all things a vehicle designed to move people from one place to another, insuring safety and security, now conveying a message suggesting that a better way to safety and security is a questionable, but sophisticated test to insure our health.

That an impersonal image, albeit one generated by high technology, could be the answer to our health care issues, is reminiscent of the hucksters who prowled frontier America. It is no different than the useless potions, often laced with alcohol or cocaine, sold to frontier Americans with the promise of improved health. This sinister, malevolent, and subliminal message is a fitting example of how modern medicine has shaken loose from the shackles of its predecessor, now offering another step towards Nirvana by way of questionable technology. In this case the lull of compliancy with a negative test or the rush to even more questionable technology with an "abnormal" test is much the same as the euphoria produced by the elixirs.

Why should that be so bothersome? Buses can and do advertise just about everything from toothpaste to safe sex. People do pay attention to these advertisements or they wouldn't be there in the first place. There doesn't appear to be any message that is too sacrosanct, certainly not personal health care issues, to find itself an advertisement on a billboard, a bus, or a subway--American capitalism at work. Many of the ads raise ethical or moral issues with respect to the message as well as the messenger. In this case where is the science to validate the claims? Has this methodology been carefully studied by medical scientists and put to the test of clinical trials? What is the motivation of the physicians who find the ad useful? The answers, of course, are no, no and the beneficiaries are the few unscrupulous radiologists, cardiologists, cardiac surgeons and the anesthesiologists who stand to prosper.

Body scans often include a "calcium count," calculated in the chest cavity, ostensibly representing coronary atherosclerosis, that is narrowing of these vessels that leads to heart attacks. If the calcium count is "abnormal" it will certainly be an invitation for more studies, including a coronary angiogram, and perhaps cardiac surgery. The question is whether patients with coronary artery disease who have the test and what follows will have better outcomes than those with the same disease without the test. It doesn't seem to make much difference to many patients who have been sold on the value of high technology and happy to get the latest technological test. Of course, we don't have the answer to the question regarding outcomes, but never mind, this scan is marketed to everyone, not necessarily those with symptoms, but to all of us. It is given the same billing as a Pap smear, a mammogram, or a cholesterol test. To join that pantheon of scientifically proven tests it would need to be validated by research, but it is not. It is a case where cleaver doctors reformulate computerized tomography to search for unproven surrogates of coronary artery disease. Since we human beings are imperfect creatures, you can bet your bottom dollar that some abnormality will be found. Mind you, all of this occurs with an asymptomatic individual who may live a long and useful life without this test or any specific intervention in spite of some degree of coronary atherosclerosis. The ad leads us to believe that this is an essential test for continued health. In fact, it is simply a strategy to substitute questionable technology for careful doctoring.

- Why do we put up with this?
- Why do we let these entrepreneurs rent free space in our brains?
- What does this have to do with rising health care costs and the promise of financial ruin for our country?
- What does all of that have to do with our health and lives?

This is the path from snake oil to misguided high technology. It is the story of greed, the way that some unprincipled physicians have continued to have their way, now with high technology, often untested, markening "elixirs of health." Instead of offering potions to unsuspecting patients, these modern day charlatans now offer unnecessary or untested procedures as a way to enhance their revenue.

Here are some facts. They are a bit dry, but important if we are to understand the problem. So, bear with me. The Office of the Actuary of the Health Care Financing Administration (HCFA) has projected that health care expenditures account for 16% of the gross domestic product and cost over 2 trillion dollars a year, with per person health spending over $7,000, and rising at a rate greater than the inflation rate. This is cause for concern. In thirty years, at this rate of increase, national health expenditures will increase to 4 trillion dollars, the cost to each American family will be $82,000 dollars, and as a society we will be unable to continue as the leader of the free world, unable to take care of our own citizens, as we fragment and head into oblivion.

At the same time physician incomes have become stagnant or have actually decreased during the past several years. According to the Center for Studying System Change (HSC), Physician incomes, after adjusting for inflation, have dropped 7% across the board during the last 10 years. This is in contradistinction to other professionals whose incomes have risen 7% during this time frame. So it looks like we are being better stewards as physicians. But wait, the devil is in the details. Physician incomes have remained at 20% of health care expenditures during the last decade. Since health care expenditures have risen to around 3 trillion dollars, 20% of three trillion is not chicken feed. The other 80% of health care expenditures, which include outpatient and in-patient hospital costs and pharmaceutical costs and which help facilitate both good and bad high technology, are also a direct result of physician ordering practices. Given that the number of procedures and sophisticated tests have increased during this time period, it becomes clearer how some unethical doctors have managed to maintain a semblance of their incomes. These unprincipled creatures have invaded high technology, have kidnapped it for their own personal use, which we will see is not altruism, but rather greed, and have become the engine driving the increased health care expenditures for reasons that this book purports to explore.

I am not suggesting that most doctors make too much money. I believe that most doctors are honorable. They are passionate about providing excellent health care, they work hard, they are devoted to their patients and to the their profession. They are a credit to the practice of medicine. The doctor who comes in during the middle of the night to deliver a baby or to pin a fractured hip is probably paid much less than his worth given the reduced stipends offered by both public and private insurers. Yet, he or she continues to do it because of commitment. Professor Uwe E. Reinhardt of Princeton writes in response to an article in the Week in Review section of The New York Times:

> In "Sending Back The Doctor's Bill" (Week in Review), you compare the incomes of American physicians with those earned by doctors in other countries and suggest that American doctors seem overpaid. A more relevant benchmark however, would seem to be the earnings of he American talent pool from which American doctors must be recruited.

Any college graduate bright enough to get into medical school surely would be able to get a high-paying job on Wall Street. The obverse is not necessarily true. Against that benchmark, every American doctor can be said to be sorely underpaid.

He goes on to say that "Physicians are the central decision makers in health care. A superior strategy might be to pay them very well for helping us reduce unwarranted health spending elsewhere". This is a central theme of this book.

The conventional wisdom, as noted above by HSC, is that the growth and development of technology is a major cause of these terrible financial facts outlined above. The Centers for Medicare and Medicaid services

(CMS) are focused on cost containment and quality improvement efforts. These are noble goals, but tinkering with the health care system, shuffling the dollars, and rationing care are little better than window dressing. These rising costs are principally due to the cascade of events that occur after unscrupulous physicians write an order, an event that is dangerously close to the epicenter of this problem. Henceforth these self-centered physicians will be identified as technophysicians. These are medical or surgical specialists who only see the color of money, whose altruism is negated or adulterated by the focus on personal gain. They have a gimmick to offer, one stanched from scientific investigation, and they substitute this for professionalism. They grab hold of a procedure, one born from science and with a legitimate use, and they subtly adjust the indications for doing this procedure in their favor, making this a profitable endeavor. This path decimates the vocational mandate of serving, caring, and altruism. These physicians are well trained, with good credentials, and aura of authenticity. But, they have bastardized their skills for unsavory goals. Technophysicians are found in all of the medical disciplines. These are the central players in the drama of rising health care expenditures.

As we closely examine the doctor-patient interface, the essential point of service in the health care industry, we come to understand how this happens. But for now, suffice it to say that it is not the growth of high technology per se that is the culprit, but rather cavalier decisions by technophysicians to use this technology, whether validated or not, when ever and where ever. This portrait includes, amongst others, the decision to carry out a complicated and dangerous operation on a fragile, elderly patient, the decision to give chemotherapy to a dying cancer patient in a futile situation, the decision to initiate hemodialysis in a situation where the patient has multiple terminal comorbidities, the decision to carry out a Caesarian section because is more convenient, the decision to apply multiple endoscopic and imaging studies to a patient with wide spread cancer where the information is next to useless, and the decision to do a mastectomy on a woman already with metastatic disease to the liver or brain. This is ground zero, these are the kind of decisions that characterize the duplicity of technophysicians.

The landscape of health care has been fundamentally altered by the recent passage of the Obama health care bill. This changes the focus somewhat and I will discuss the impact this will have on conventional private medicine, the challenge to private health care, and a meaningful response to the gauntlet that has been thrown. But for now, the task is to trace the origin of this monster, this obscene embrace of high technology by some doctors, which I submit is a major cause of the dysfunctional and broken American health care system.

The origin of this financial monster, this broken health care system, lays embedded within the evolutionary events of American medicine during the past 50 years. However, let's turn the clock back further. The concept of dualism, namely the nature of man separated into body and soul, dates back thousands of years, but it was during the period of the enlightenment when western philosophers began to critically study body and soul and where the foundation for dualism was laid. As the age of faith came to a close, men began to question long held dogma regarding the nature of things: the heliocentric universe, gravity, the circulation of blood, as well as the spatial configuration of earth. The age of faith became a casualty of the age of reason. Philosophers struggled to reconcile the soul, the domain of thought processes, and the center of emotion, with the workings of the human body. Scientists found themselves preoccupied with unraveling secrets of the cosmos, the underpinnings of an emerging physical science, ultimately describing a human body whose functions worked automatically, like a clock, with clock-like precision, and seemingly independent of thought, state of mind, dreams, or any discernable metaphysical influence. It was as if a master craftsman had designed man, wound him up like a clock, and let him go. This was the period of time that gave us Darwin, Copernicus, Newton, Voltaire, Shakespeare, Adam Smith, John Locke, and Rene Descartes. It was Descartes, a 17 century philosopher, who led the effort to understand the totality of the mind and body. Finally, perhaps out of frustration, he separated the two, postulating that man's body worked independent of his mind and thoughts. Thus, health simply required restoring or preserving the clockwork of man's body without paying much attention to man's thoughts, emotions, or soul. Other than repairing the clock, there was no need for intellectual inquiry, new knowledge, or new information about the totality of man. The noted Harvard philosopher, Alfred North Whitehead, has identified this bifurcation of nature as the cause of misguided medical inquiry adversely affecting education of physicians and the practice of medicine in our time. We will have more to say about that.

At the same time theological leaders struggled to understand the nature of man, given new scientific discoveries, striving to leave a place for God, a celestial connection, preserving the legacy of the Church. Their consternation was that thinkers stopped asking philosophical questions about the nature of life, the nature of man, God's purpose in creation, and man's purpose in life; rather, they watched in dismay as these great enlightenment thinkers and leaders drifted towards the physical sciences: mathematics, navigation, astronomy, agriculture, and medicine. The scientific method was born; a systematic manner to try and understand the world we live in. The scientific method required the careful observation of phenomena and the development of an hypothesis, a causal mechanism for the phenomena. To validate this hypothesis, so that it could be used to predict other phenomena, experimentation was required. This is where the rub came in; scientists needed physical experiments to make this work. The results of these experiments needed to be tangible and reproducible, without bias. The scientific method paved the way for these new thinkers to successfully understand many observable phenomena, and later phenomena less well observable. Enlightenment thinkers were seduced by an impersonal devotion to the scientific method, relegating the mystery of life to scientifically uncharted territory, simply awaiting the moment when science would explain all. The somewhat conceited supposition was that scientific discoveries, in the aggregate, would eventually add up to a supreme knowledge regarding the nature of life.

Contemporary medical science dates its birth to this era. The new medical scientists satisfied themselves with the study of the structure and function of Homo sapiens as a means for maintaining and restoring health. Man's soul, brain, and emotions were not worthy of scientific inquiry and did not play a pivotal role in health and disease. From the 17th century until the 21st century, answers to human illness have continued to be found as an outcome from scientific investigation.

Gradually and imperceptibly the notion of illness, gave way to the concept of disease, a limited, definable event, the result of linear causality, and amenable to cure. Illness, as opposed to disease, does not speak to the afflictions of man as a machine, but rather dis ease of the soul, where suffering is consequent to man assuming ultimate and complete control, a dislocation from a higher power, where individual will power is found wanting. Suffering, a consequence of this spiritual dislocation, manifests as chronic pain, insomnia, malaise, loneliness, fear, anorexia, weight loss and depression. Some of this falls within the discipline of mental illness, but it is more. This dislocation of the soul is much more apparent now with chronic illnesses and to that extent medical science should be applauded for providing us with longevity. Medical scientists have dressed up these afflictions with fancy names, i.e. chronic fatigue syndrome, fibromyalgia, irritable bowel syndrome, cyclic vomiting syndrome, and melancholy. By limiting themselves to the standard allopathic approach, that is the approach which embraces the scientific method, the results have not been good. Terminal illness is not seen worthy of hope, pain is ameliorated with narcotics, depression is swept aside with psycho pharmacy, and functional illnesses, a euphemism for dis ease, have become the substrate for unnecessary, costly, and dangerous technology, a circumstance whereby technophysicians take advantage of the situation.

As scientists wrestled with the notion of disease, the function and dysfunction of the human body were found in smaller and smaller units of the body. Disease resulted from some outside cause that which led to direct effects on the circuitry of our bodies. The scientific method was endorsed as the only valid way to discover this dysfunction and the cause of human disease. All research and all the advances in medical knowledge have occurred from that time to the present embracing these principles. Matters of the mind, the soul, and dislocation were caste aside. The rub is that this scientific methodology has worked well, especially during the first half of the 20th century when infectious and nutritional diseases were conquered. But wait. Not so with chronic diseases, which have occupied center stage during that second half of the 20th century until now, and these have played a significant role in this drama of rising health costs. The reality is that the scientific method seems to work less well with many chronic diseases, begging the question of the applicability of the scientific method in this instance. Many of these patients are now seeking help from alternative medicine. Naturopathy, homeopathy, acupuncture, and intuitive practitioners now account for significant out of pocket health care dollars because they will at least listen to patients with chronic pain, chronic fatigue, irritable bowel syndrome, and any number of so-called functional illness. Technophysicians are be quick to see these patients if they have a gimmick or procedure to offer.

For the past 75 years physicians have been trained to understand health and disease from this Cartesian point of view. The medical school curricula embodies this format, research occurs embracing this principle, advancements occur limited to this vantage point. The structure and function of our bodies, the nature of the subcellular elements, from the nucleus of a cell to the genetic code embodied within DNA, are all outgrowths of the scientific method. This same scientific method has led to the development of wonderful technology including ventilation machines, extra-corporeal pumps to support the circulation during cardiac surgery, renal dialysis technology, and organ transplants. Today, molecular biology is the quintessence of the scientific method as applied to medicine. Although the distance from the bench to the bedside has increased, that is, the applicability of research is less discernable, there have been a number of new and important molecular biological discoveries: understanding tissue rejection with the promise of improved organ transplantation, an improved understanding of autoimmune diseases, unraveling the inflammatory process, the human genome project and the future treatment of genetic disease, and the molecular messengers which are involved in the transformation of normal cells to malignant cells.

There is certainly nothing wrong with all of this. But these wonderful advances have spawned medical technology, some elegant and well tested, others less well tested, and this technology has fallen into the hands of technophysicians, the chief culprits of our dysfunctional health system.

So it has been with medicine during the past fifty years. We have concentrated our efforts on repairing the disordered clock, leaving in limbo the soul, the animus, that unique force which makes us human. Psychiatry is actively engaged with the elements of chronic illness, but psychiatrist's stipends pale in significance to that of technophysicians. So while their efforts are to be lauded, mental health spending is not the cause of rising health care costs. Something is wrong! In spite of rising health care costs our overall health report card is not good and I submit that technophysicians are much of the problem.

The birth of US hospitals occurred towards the end of the 19th century with the marriage of anesthesia and surgery. Prior to that our hospitals were primarily for the mentally ill. With the growth of hospitals health care became more complex, costs became an issue, and out of this milieu was born the medical insurance industry. Initially, the methodology of the fledgling insurance companies was a fee-for-service format, an indemnity formula, whereby the premiums, often picked up by employers, provided a healthy margin for the insurance companies and covered the medical fees for those patients who could afford the premiums. Health care costs were much lower after World War II and insurance found it profitable to sell plans with affordable premiums. There were fewer tests, fewer procedures, patients were comfortable with a stay in the hospital, where bed rest was the major cost, but the growth of technology and the birth of technophysicians was right around the corner. 1965 was a watershed period and profound changes occurred with the enactment of Medicare and Medicaid legislation. The federal government landed on the beachhead, first with Medicare and Medicaid, and ultimately with a heavy foot in the health care machinery, with future strings attached to future allocations. At first, the fee-for-service format for doctor's services and hospitals was used by the government, but when costs continued to rise, often the result of abuse by technophysicians, other insurance methods were created. Technology continued to grow. Congress was acutely aware of the steep rise in health care costs during the Nixon administration and during the 1970s HMO (Health Maintenance Organizations) legislation was written, heavily influenced by the Kaiser experience. By 1980 HMOs were springing up in various markets. During this decade Congress enacted the hospital DRG (Disease Related Groupings) program that provided a lump sum of money to the hospital, which now found itself in an uneasy contract with the government. This was purported to cover the total care of a hospitalized patient with whatever disease, described by a disease-related group or category, reigning in the hospitals obscene spending which was closely tied to the activity of their technophysicians.

Hospitals found themselves cut off, no more horn of plenty, the faucet was turned off, and administrators scampered to convert from a productivity-based economy to a cost control based economy. The goal was to reduce physician-ordered tests, procedures, surgeries, and to cut the length of stay in the hospital. A faint fault line developed between hospitals and doctors.

Technology continued to grow and health care costs continued to rise. As a result managed care was born, nursed by the government, and fondled by private insurance companies, to take a shot at controlling the costs. Using the HMO format, insurance companies, both for profit and non profit, including Medicare and Medicaid, capitated payment to providers (a euphemism for doctors); that is, a lump sum was prepaid per patient per year to cover all of the medical costs of patients subscribed in the plans. If the physician-generated costs were above this amount then the physician was at risk and money needed to come out of his pocket. This is essentially why physicians have formed into groups; to manage cost and risk. Or, if not capitated, managed care organizations offered salaries to doctors employed by HMOs, which attempt to control how many patients are seen or how many procedures are performed. Both of these schemes have been abused by technophysicians. This abuse was related to unnecessary procedures, like CT scans for headaches, or feeding tubes for terminally ill patients, primarily because technophysicians broadened the indications for intervention, substituting volume for the decreased reimbursement rates, and substituting avarice for case selection. Thus, health care costs have continued to rise, ultimately driving up our national health care expenditures.

The question of why this is so is central to this discussion of the health care crisis and is linked to three economic realities: the bifurcation of science and technology, the gulf that has developed between those costs born by the insurance industry and what we patients actually pay, and the cost of educating a physician. Technophysicians are the common denominator. As a group, they have been given birth by this cauldron, leavened by one or all of these three economic realities. (1) The technological tools of scientists were bequeathed to specialty physicians, but ultimately snatched up by technophysicians, who were able to drive up their fees, with a spinoff to hospitals, who owned the equipment and also got a big piece of the action. (2) We patients have become more and more isolated from the realities of health care costs because of the various insurance schemes and we are insulated from the realities of the escalating expenditures. As a group, a group that represents the total national interest, we have had precious little feel for what it costs to have a procedure or an operation, or to be hospitalized with all that goes on during that experience. Itemized bills are frequently misleading as cost shifting obfuscates reality. Hospitals have no problem charging a hefty fee for an aspirin tablet, shifting costs in a way that confuses the payer and patient. We take for granted that we are covered. The rise in our co-payments, which insurance companies have found economically advantageous, has increased our awareness, but it is still feeble, as the itemized bill is laden with arcane terms. If the hospital experience is covered, the need to scrutinize an itemized bill is less because human nature trumps the need to know. This is the second major player in the health care crisis; naiveté and ignorance about these rising costs. (3) The costs of education for today's medical student are in great measure due to the costs of purchasing high technology equipment. If this equipment was used by proper, ethical medical or surgical specialists, less would be needed and the costs would be less, simply because there would be fewer physicians wanting to be specialists because the driving force would be ethical case selection rather than the low hanging fruit sought out by the technophysicians. But, that is not the case. Technophysicians have increased in numbers exponentially, shifting much of the teaching of medicine towards technomedicine. Thus all physicians entering private practice at the present time have outstanding debts in the same category as a home mortgage, i.e. between $100,000 and $200,000, thanks to the technophysicians. There is much more incentive to gravitate towards being a technophysician since the money is good. This is the third player in the present health care crisis.

Medical school faculty have found that seeing patients, who were now amply covered by the new governmental insurance plans, provided an additional revenue stream for medical schools and academic health care centers, which were just beginning to feel reduced funding from the federal government. Faculty participation in patient care and faculty involvement with technology became the cash cow, covering the deficits as federal funds for research and teaching could not keep pace with growth. This is where the tools of the technophysician have germinated, where valid technology is misused for personal gain. This is where technophysicians learn how to subordinate health care is to avarice.

To recapitulate, these three players: the bifurcation of technology from science, the isolation of patients from true health care costs, and the exorbitant debt born by today's new physician, account for much of the maelstrom from which the health care crisis has arisen. These three are interrelated and must be seen this way as we explore their individual and combined effect on rising health care expenditures and our health care crisis. For instance, the cost of educating a medical or surgical specialist, a group from which technophysicians are born, inevitably affects the average debt burden of medical school graduates. This cost has risen dramatically because of the costs attendant to high technology. New doctors gravitate towards technomedicine for financial reasons. The obscure nature of the pricing of medical services makes it easier for technophysicians to influence these rising health care expenditures and contribute to the mess. But again, the driving force is the technophysician, who masquerades as a specialty physician. Patients have been sold and accepted the fact that technology represents science and that they can expect to be part of the victory of science over disease. These are fallacies often promulgated by technophysicians: namely, that technology equals science and that science will ultimately conquer disease.

All of this might be tolerable if the facts revealed that we had the best health in the world, that our longevity was tops, that there was significant success in dealing with chronic disease, and that our senior citizens were more productive than the rest of the world; then one could argue that the price of technophysicians, might be worth it. But they don't! If we could point to the success of technophysicians in expanding access to our health care system to all segments of society, making health care more affordable and more available to every American, providing more insight with respect to the cause and cure of chronic diseases, then the price of high tech might be worth it. But we can't!

Our societal health report card is not good. Here are some interesting and disturbing facts. The World Health Report 2000, *Health Systems: Improving Performance,* ranked the U.S. health care system 37th in the world. When compared with the other industrialized nations of the world, our infant mortality rate is 39th, , our adult female mortality rate is 43rd, our adult male mortality is 42nd, and our life expectancy is 36th. This must be seen with the backdrop of the U.S. being number one in terms of health care spending per capita.

We Americans now spend nearly 30 billion dollars out of pocket for alternative health care, which includes chiropractic, naturopathic medicine, acupuncture, intuitive medicine, and homeopathy. This is in great measure because of dissatisfaction with our allopathic health system. We spend over three trillion dollars per year on medical expenditures, yet there are still 40 million of us without insurance, fellow citizens who have jobs, yet making too much money to qualify for Medicaid and too little for health insurance. There are 40 million additional citizens who are woefully underinsured with very limited access to our gargantuan health care system. Yet, in an emergency these underinsured individuals do get treated, usually in overworked hospital emergency rooms, albeit minimal treatment at times, and this cost is born by all of us, further driving up national health care costs.

This is a major problem.

Heretofore, government has been unable to control the escalating costs. Those 160 million who are insured represent those of us who are asleep at the switch. Politicians don't mess with this group because they are satisfied. Should they be? No. This group's passive acquiescence to their physician's recommendations is interpreted as a tacit approval of the expansion of technophysicians. This group, which represents most of us, has bought in to undeserved faith. The glitter and promises of high technology are a soothing and misleading tonic, providing technophysicians with a masque. With the recent heath care reform bill, which is now law, the 160 million who have private insurance and at risk, is the group that needs to refocus and help make changes necessary for a vibrant and competitive private heath care response.

Why should we care? What does all of this have to do with our lives? Isn't this someone else's problem? What could I possibly do about all of this? As long as insurance pays for the stuff what difference does all of this make? And now, nearly all citizens are guaranteed access, aided by government subsidies, further blurring the real causes and solution for this debacle. But there is still time if we Americans awaken to these facts. Our private health care system is at risk, but we citizens still have time right the ship of state I will have more to say about that.

This begs the question of what is the relationship of this silly CT scan ad to the American health care delivery system and to the industrial-medical complex, which finds itself in a sinister vortex, heading for catastrophe. It is obviously not just the body CT scan, but rather the cavalier and aggressive way that technophysicians are contributing the problem.

Health care in America is headed towards disaster. This is not to say that we do not have a remarkable health care system, only that the costs have risen so dramatically during the past 30 years, continue to rise in spite of managed care, and at the present rate promise national bankruptcy within the next 30 years. Now, solvency has been given a shot in the arm, with a huge national price tag, and quality stands to suffer. The CT scan is part of the problem that creates runaway health care expenditures, which is short on quality, but has provided significant profits for technophysicians. This may all seem abstract and irrelevant, but the consequences of inadequate and substandard health care for our children should be a wake up call.

It is important to note that this is not the result of the government, the HMOs or insurance industry, the pharmaceutical or health care manufacturing industry, the legal profession, or any other bit player. The finger points at us, the consumer, who have gone to sleep at the switch, who have slumbered while technophysicians have jacked up the cost of health care for reasons that have more to do with their well being than our health. It is we, the consumer, who have abrogated our responsibility, and accepted hook, line, and sinker, the notion that modern technology can promise us immortality and freedom from pain and suffering. When we accept that notion, we fall right into the hands of techophysicians.

What can we do about this problem? There is no quick fix. Yet, without change we face either national bankruptcy or some variation of national health. We are already heading down the path towards national health. Our choices seem to be either succumbing to big brother, giving the government more and more discretionary power over our lives as it attempts to control costs, or to sit back, fiddling while Rome burns, fighting terrorism, and losing the battle on the home front as we slide into national bankruptcy. Big government can promise universal coverage and public financing, as well as rid ourselves of technophysicians, but at the expense of quality, leaving all of us is the grips of mediocrity, with limited expectations, and virtually no exposure to the process of healing. We must be careful not to throw the baby out with the wash. High technology is here to stay. With proper case selection, buttressed by ethics and morality, it is a major step forward for quality health care. Quality will be discussed later, but for now we must be certain that we leave room for altruistic high technology physicians.

Government cannot replace, replicate, or infuse those elements of healing that emanate from a meaningful relationship between a doctor and his patient. Caring, support, and empathy are difficult, if not impossible to measure, but I submit that most patients intuitively know when these are missing in their relationship with a physician. My own experience leads me to believe that these elements are usually missing with technophysicians. These intangibles will not result from government intervention, where the goal is affordable premiums, universal coverage, and rationing. The government will never be able to instill a quest for improved quality, nor the elements of ethics and morality. This will only happen when physicians who work at the point of service understand the problem and make changes themselves.

We citizens need to become involved. We need to understand the problem and roll up our shirt sleeves. No one can do that for us in a meaningful way. In the following pages I attempt to share my experiences and provide evidence for my indictment of technophysicians. My hope is that with proper information a public dialogue will occur, not government sponsored, not industry funded, but a public dialogue leading to a public demand that changes need to be made in the education of physicians. The task is to identify the locus where this has all gone wrong. The next chapter explores the landscape and focuses on the central point of dysfunction.

Chapter 2
The Power Of The Pen A Switch That Galvanizes An Industry

Sheets of rain fell torrentially across the windshield of his aging Mazda. The rivulets of moisture distorted the light from on-coming vehicles creating a surreal dimension. Robert Munoz, a veteran of thirty years, the recipient of a purple heart and a bronze metal for his efforts in Viet Nam, was now gripped with more fear and apprehension than he could recall during the Tet Offensive. Robert Munoz was a friend of mine. I met him while serving in the Army in Germany as a medical officer during the Vietnam war. His story sent chills up my spine. He had always had difficulty managing his weight, but now, without even trying, he had lost nearly 10 pounds. It was the constant pain in his abdomen that was most bothersome. He had been single for three years since the tragic death of his wife in an automobile accident. His children were grown and living on the East Coast. There was no family with whom to share his fears, and he had fears. He recalled caring for his father who had died a slow and painful death from cancer of the pancreas and this was not lost on the moment.

Traffic was moving slowly, too slowly for someone who was finally going to keep the appointment he had made with this new doctor. Doctors were not his favorite breed, not a type of person he had relished visiting, demanding that he make his body available for an examination, assuming that he would make himself vulnerable. Not this Special Forces First Sergeant. Not this battle-tested warrior carrying wounds from mortal combat. He recalled his wife admonishing him to reconsider that attitude, to take better care of himself, to listen to professional advice. Those words, plus the increasing pain, were the only reasons why he picked up the phone and made the damn appointment. He finally made a left turn into the parking lot, rain pouring and obscuring his view, and with some trepidation, he parked his car. Getting out, shielding himself from the deluge, and walking the few steps to the front door of the office were as tedious and frightening as being on patrol in the Central Highlands. He could feel the enemy following his every step, intuitively sensing the proximity of deadly land mines. But, his mission was clear. He had to heed to his wife's advice and get some relief from the pain. The waiting room chairs were squeaky and uncomfortable. The room was full of elderly patients, mothers with crying babies, and sullen teenagers picking their noses, fidgeting, and arguing with their mothers. What was he doing there? Why put up with all this shit? His mind raced back in time, to 1971, the military hospital in Saigon, and the pain he had felt in his thigh from a bullet wound, guys laying around him in various degrees of discomfort. The smell of blood, infection, and disinfectants all blended together, forever fixed in his memory. The military nurses were changing his dressing, readjusting the position of his leg, a hand on his shoulder for comfort.

No, that's not what he felt. It was an elderly lady whose skeletal hand was gently shaking his shoulder, trying to direct his attention to the nurse who was now calling for him to move into the examining room. He jolted, a bit startled, but moved toward the nurse and into the room. The smell of disinfectant teased his memory, the featureless examining table became the enemy, and time morphed into an endless stream of recollections, an interminable amount of time, until the doctor casually meandered into the examining room. There was an indifferent introduction, a limp handshake, and a slight nod of the head, which was interpreted as an invitation to get on the examining table.

The doctor asked, "what's the matter?" never actually looking him in the eye. There was no warmth, no invitation to be part of the moment. He took a deep breath, muttered a silent prayer, and began to recount his problems. As best he could, he recounted the chronology of his symptoms, relating the onset of the pain, a tingling feeling over the skin of his abdomen, but before he could finish, the doctor was redirecting the conversation, launching a salvo of bland questions, none of which Munoz could actually remember, and within an instant the doctor pulled a beautiful Mount Blanc pen from the pocket of his flowing white coat. As he muttered something unintelligible, the doctor put pen to paper;

fancy stationary embossed with elegance. The doctor's physical exam was cursory at best. Munoz actually wanted him to look at a peculiar rash he had on his abdomen, but the doctor simply listened to his heart and lungs with his stethoscope placed over his shirt. In an instant he casually wrote orders, which would launch Sergeant Munoz on one more mission. With no protestation, Munoz had relinquished his freedom, this battletested warrior, to an industry which now had him in its grasp, to this citadel of modern medicine, which he had been led to believe was interested in his welfare. Munoz needed more time, more information from the doctor, he felt intimidated, not invited to tell his story. He felt like an insignificant part of a well choreographed event that seemed to leave him out. It was only later that learned that he did not have cancer, it was a case of shingles, a diagnosis that the doctor should have been able to make from the examining table, by simply inspecting the skin of his abdomen. But the doctor didn't look, his exam was as casual as his demeanor, simply a hand on Sergeant Munoz' abdomen without having him remove his shirt. And for that, the health care industry was activated and another patient's sanctity was violated, leaving disgust in its wake, but profits for the industry and a patient confused because all of his fancy tests were in fact normal. It was only when he went to the VA clinic and he found a physician who seemed to care, who carefully listened without interrupting Sgt. Munoz, and the diagnosis was made.

A physician's pen generates nearly 70% of health care costs. It is these same costs that are rising at such a rapid rate that the solvency of our health care system, not to mention that of the nation, is placed in jeopardy. The physician's pen. This insignificant writing instrument, this highly refined modification of man's earliest attempt to record events, is all that stands between any physician, but most particularly a technophysician, and the unleashing of an insatiable healthcare industry, a tidal wave of activity, a stream of closely connected events that promise cost but cannot insure quality. It happened to sergeant Munoz. All of us are potential cannon fodder. Higher cost usually implies increased quality, except when it comes to medical care. This is the crux of the problem. Munoz was like so many of us; overwhelmed with the moment, not knowing what to say or do, afraid to look stupid, not willing to ask pertinent questions. For a soldier, discipline and rank require obedience, but even with civilians, technophysicians leave very little room for a full discussion. Technophysicians are in a hurry, the trappings of authority are suffocating, the language of doctors is indecipherable. Munoz, like most patients, assumed that his well being was paramount. This is not always the case, but without asking, how are we to know what is right? Patients like Munoz are invited to trust their physician's ministrations, and most of the time patients can. But, technophysicians often subtly shift the shades of truth in a way that their recommendations seem inviolable. We patients feel relegated to acquiescence.

Early in their training, we young physicians learn how to write orders with our pens. This honored tradition serves as our passport to autonomy. We grind these orders out day and night, in the midst of bedlam and peril, whether or not our motives are pure, whether or not our thinking is clear, whether or not our agenda is honorable. As I reflect in my own lifetime and my own journey I have seen where order writing has led to mistakes that seem to tumble upon themselves, exacerbating the situation, leading to results that cause other perturbations, all following the initial written order. This process of writing orders provides baleful background music to an industry that seems to be sewing the seeds of its own demise.

The learning process is so innocent. Insulated from societal realities, we young doctors follow the advice of our mentors and tuck the methodology away in our left brain. Physician orders deal with patient comfort issues, life sustaining measures, the monitoring of tasks, and the ordering of tests. Tests are the venue where the initial embrace with high technology takes place, an initiation into the mystery and magic of angiography, fibreoptics, magnetic resonance and laser phototherapy. For Munoz it would be a CT scan of his abdomen, an ultrasound of his gall bladder and endoscopy by his gastroenterologist. But these decisions were made without a careful history, an inadequate physical exam, all without inviting much input from Munoz. This left him more apprehensive than when he initially walked into the doctor's office. At times the first doctor we see is a generalist, a general practitioner, an internist, or an emergency room doctor. The odds are, however, that we will eventually be shuttled to a specialist, who may or may not be trustworthy, and the cacophony of order writing becomes overwhelming, blurring the moment, leaving patients, like Munoz, in a subordinate position, a no win proposition. This is not right. I believe that patients need to part of the process, part of an active dialogue, not just a supplicant. My own experience with the trappings of high tech medicine leave little room for the patient's active participation.

Orders written are communicated to nurses and other ancillary providers to start the ball rolling. Patients are admitted to the hospital, to the ICU, to a nursing home. Nurses are instructed how often to check the patient, how often to get vital signs, when and what blood tests to draw, what x-rays to obtain, what medicines to give, and what procedures to prepare for and anticipate. It is all very organized and well inscribed into the hospital lexicon. With a flick of the wrist, an industry is switched on; an industry whose rising costs portend major problems. This remarkable discretionary power handed to us physicians is predicated upon the axiom that they we been properly trained and that the patient's welfare is the primary agenda. Unfortunately, during my career this has often not been the case. Rather, this discretionary power predictably activates the health care industry, which is often insensitive and foreboding, substituting an automatic pilot approach for intimacy. All one needs to do is to walk into any major hospital and see the lines of patients awaiting a procedure, alone and frightened. My take of hospitals is that they have become hi tech citadels, substituting machines for compassion, more focused on tests and procedures than comfort, interested in getting patients in and out as quickly as possible.

The pen literally dances across the physician's order sheet and the industrial-medical complex is given life. Huge medical megalopolises are born from the ink; new technologies are acquired; new layers of governmental bureaucracy evolve to control the technology; hospital systems rush to merge in an effort to manage the cost control measures which flow from the regulators. The industry's latticework becomes more and more complex, a maze. I have seen this happen from the vantage point of the Chief of Staff of a large California hospital.

If the agenda is something other than quality, if decisions are thoughtless, if they are made for self-serving reasons, then the power of that pen is adulterated and dangerous. It becomes an instrument for the perpetuation of the health-care crisis. I believe that this is ground zero, where the health care crisis has germinated and is perpetuated.

We doctors learn to pull this puppy out from the pocket of our white coats, scrubs, or dress shirts, and scribble away. There is a rush, a feeling of power, suddenly on stage, center court. We physicians deftly leave our imprint on a moment, on an industry, on mankind. The medical profession has ensured that no one else has the power to make a medical decision, that only we physicians can write orders. In every state in the Union laws place what is medically necessary in the hands and pen of physicians.

Woven within the fabric of the order sheet are issues that deal with the meaning of life, the definition of life, the role of the patient, and the physician's agenda. In a crisis patients often search for spiritual answers, a longing for compassion. Patients need more than a hastily calculated prognosis. There is the need to know how this illness might change their lives, how it will affect their relationships, jobs, future, and what they can do to be a participant in healing. For example, it is more that simply giving penicillin for pneumonia. There is a need to know how the pneumonia happened, will it happen again, is there some underlying propensity, will lungs be permanently damaged, what can be done to prevent another episode. None of this is readily apparent. The mechanics of order writing often obfuscate these issues. But, the issues are present, ready to be seen if there is interest. In those early idealistic medical school years the welfare of the patient was first and foremost. During internships and residencies, some of the idealism is attenuated. We young physician learn shortcuts, ways to embrace the linear, reductionist, causality system. We become a disciple of allopathic medicine and in time, vaguely aware of how the pharmaceutical industry is turned on, how the manufacture of health care hardware is energized, how insurance companies and HMOs are born, how health care executives, politicians, health care engineers, and lawyers are given life by our orders which are subtly nurtured by our own philosophy. So much is at stake.

As a young house officer, writing orders was an instant high, a heady rush, promising control and authority. It never occurred to me that the industry shrugged ever so slightly, responding with a plethora of high technology, when orders were written. The myriad tasks generated by my orders were out of sight. I was oblivious to the financial impact created by my order writing. The cost of tests, drugs, consultation, and procedures were obscured by a false sense of propriety.

The Munoz story, the underlying motif of incomplete doctoring, is readily apparent in other circumstances. Melissa White was a young woman with diabetes. She was a juvenile diabetic who required insulin shots and who had been suffering with this problem for several years. As part of any residency program, physicians were trained to select the proper dose and frequency of insulin, adjusting for any number of variables, as well ensure that the patient is taught how to determine their blood sugar and how to administer the insulin. Patients are taught how to draw up the necessary amount of insulin into a syringe. They are taught how to inject themselves. When I was in training patients learned the technique by practicing on a orange, the peel being a surrogate for skin, giving the patient a sense of the depth and feel of an injection The orders written for Ms. White were very explicit, including a sliding scale of insulin calculated for the amount of sugar determined in her blood. This was very important information for the patient and her family. In spite of what was felt to be clear-cut orders, Melissa White was readmitted to the hospital over and over with diabetic ketoacidosis, a condition characterized by dehydration, kidney failure, often leading to coma and death. These problems occur when the amount of insulin is inadequate and the patient's blood sugar is inordinately high. The reason for her readmission time and time again was due to her diabetes being out of control. It was a mystery. The discharge orders reflected her insulin needs based upon her diet, her weight, and other medical conditions. She seemed to understand the gravity of the situation each time she was discharged. A conference was finally called with the supervising physician, Melissa, her case manager and her mother. What could be wrong here? She was carefully walked through her calculation and administration of insulin. Her mother assured all present that she understood how to calculate her insulin dose and when and how to administer it. The mother proudly recounted every detail, including how fresh oranges were bought each week for the purpose of injecting the insulin. What? How could this be? Injecting the orange? As a young doctor I could not believe this was happening. The temptation is to blame the patient, or the dietician. This was a learning experience for me, learning that when an order is written there needs to be some accountability on the part of the physician, who in this instance was me, who was, after all, the only one who could write an order, which is presumably after careful thinking and consideration. Making certain that the order is carried out properly is one of the tasks of order writing. Order writing is very powerful. Patients and nurses count on their veracity. When doctors are less than focused, disasters occur and that is exactly what happened to Melissa. It was assumed that she understood that the orange peel was a training tool. How could this happen? There are any number of possibilities, not the least of which may have been that the patient and/her mother were not attentive. In this case her insulin had mostly been given intravenously when she was admitted in a gravely ill situation. On each occasion, as she improved, the insulin was converted to the subcutaneous route, but it was given by the nurses without her having been given a chance to participate. These were orders given by we physicians and dutifully carried out by the nurses, incomplete orders without the opportunity for Melissa to become part of the process. The buck has to stop somewhere, physicians guard their precious order writing status, they earned it, but inattention to order writing can lead to catastrophes, which nearly happened.

James T. Hansen, M.D.

Order writing has evolved from an art form, into an event highly regulated and scrutinized; yet, still solely a physician activity. Orders are a source of concern in the out patient arena, but it is within the hospital environment that they cause such mischief. With the marriage of surgical technique to anesthesia, hospitals became the center of the new American medical cosmos. It was to the hospitals that doctors gravitated. It followed that admitting a patient to a hospital separated that person from his normal environment, and at the same time facilitated the separation of the disease from the person. We physicians sold the public on the notion that if you don't feel well, a hospital bed is the best place to be. We physicians convinced our patients that a short stay in the hospital was the most expeditious way to get tested and treated. The milieu for serious order writing took shape.

Hospitals are very expensive places, at times understaffed, and a threat to one's health if you consider that nosocomial infections are a major cause of hospital deaths. The new paradigm has been to shift most health care to the ambulatory side of the equation, reducing hospital length of stays, and directing patients to surgicenters for relatively minor procedures. But even these arenas become the target of physician order writing.

Hospital admissions are now more highly scrutinized, especially in markets highly penetrated by managed care. But, inappropriate admissions continue and are a function of ill-advised physician orders. Patients are admitted with chest pain, fever, anemia, diarrhea, back pain, and weight loss by their private physicians or by emergency room physicians because of extraneous pressures from family, because of physician uncertainty, because of a physician's boiler-plate behavior, or to help justify the use of expensive technology. These are not patients who need high acuity nursing and close monitoring. They are admitted for reasons known only to the physician, but reasons often made without careful thought.

As a Chief of Staff I have seen how writing orders to move a patient from an acute bed to a critical care unit is another oft-abused activity. Patients who are terminal, whose medical situations are futile, who have critical lab values but otherwise stable, do not need a critical care unit. It makes no sense to place a patient with a "do not resuscitate" order in a critical care unit where the focus is to use whatever is necessary to save a life. But it's done every day and I have done it. In my experience at least ten percent of the ICU patients on any given day do not need to be there. This ten percent stands apart from those patients awaiting transfer to a lower acuity bed. The cost of intensive care units is prohibitive and one example of quality in health care not predictably made better with increased cost.

One of the major logjams has been placing chronically ill patients into nursing homes or other step-down units. Many of these patients would be better off at home, with loved ones, but as a society we have come to believe that illness means hospitalization. Not infrequently we physicians have inappropriately displaced family in favor of hospitalization, subtly replacing family responsibility with a noisy, brightly lit, impersonal in-patient substitution, promising mostly unhappiness, and profits. Special diets, frequent vital signs, low flow oxygen, expensive medications, and complicated nursing tasks drive up the costs. Some of these orders are written a certain way because that was the way the physician was trained. We physicians receive our training in large, tertiary, teaching hospitals, where the patients are very sick, and require a different approach. Out of habit, physicians continue to write a myriad of orders, some inappropriate, without much thought, because that is the way we always did it.

Medication orders are routinely abused. We physicians are in the pharmaceutical industry's back pocket. The most expensive and the newest drug is the one often chosen, perhaps because of audacity or an over inflated sense of control. Dosage patterns are often suspect, the physician using more or less than necessary, at time because of our own ignorance, adding to costs and complications. Clinical pharmacists and clever nurses are very helpful in these situations, but technophysicians are often loath to take their advice, perhaps a perceived broach of their authority. Pharmacists and nurses are often too busy to lend a hand.

Ordering specialized tests and procedures goes hand and hand with being in a hospital. Just being hospitalized often adversely affects judgment as to the necessity of a procedure; the technology is so available it's difficult to resist. It was certainly hard for me to resist. The marriage between hospitals and hi-technology makes this a hazardous place for many who either do not need hi-tech, or could have it done more carefully and conveniently as an outpatient. The decision to operate is more easily made if the patient is already hospitalized. If a high-tech procedure or surgical procedure is indicated, yet not an emergency, technophysicians are reluctant to discharge the patient to home, perhaps because it poses an inconvenience, perhaps because of clinical uncertainty, or perhaps because of a fear that our patient might not return.

This same physician's pen is the instrument that unlocks the world of high technology to many unsuspecting patients. With the stroke of the pen the rules of the game are changed. The effort to heal a patient, which by necessity includes the totality of the human condition and the notion of suffering, is something quite different from the goals of high technology which are to reorder our circuitry from a reductionist point of view, with an eye towards curing. The notion of curing often leaves the patient bewildered, without understanding, with emotional uncertainty. The essence of healing is something quite different; it includes listening, translating, and interpretation. This is the calling of the clinician that treats illness and not just disease, the antithesis of the type of physician who thinks in a linear fashion, seeking out causality, fixing the broken clock. Not only is the patient left bewildered, but it drives up the cost. Not only the cost of high technology, which many times is unnecessary, but the door is left open for patient readmissions because the experience has been incomplete, the patient's questions have not been properly answered, expectations have not been clarified, and the promise of outpatient support is feeble.

I am reminded of an African-American attorney who complained to me about the care she had received at the hospital where I was the Chief-of-Staff. Denise Williams was a heavy set, powerful, black woman, who had carved out a new life after her husband of 20 years divorced her. After law school she became a very successful personal injury lawyer which, of course, provided added weight to her complaints.

She had been having chest pain for several months. She had learned to manage her life without any outside help, so to seek medical aid was a surrender of sorts. She finally took herself to our emergency room, which she described as impersonal and chaotic, and after waiting longer than she liked, she was seen by a harried, overworked, cynical, ruffled physician, who after a cursory examination and with the stoke of his pen, had her admitted and made ready for a cardiac consultation. She remembered very little of the rushed and complicated ER conversation, but she did remember sitting on a table, scantily clothed, a torn paper gown partially covering her chest, one breast nearly uncovered, feeling discounted and vulnerable. She was afraid to ask questions, something she did well as an attorney, feeling overwhelmed by the symphony of fellow patients moaning, crying, and screaming. But she had enough presence of mind to recount to the ER physician that the pain was first noted when working out at the gym. When she told the ER doctor that her father had died from a heart attach, she was immediately admitted. The ER doctor said that he was worried about her heart, which was understandable. Her electrocardiogram was non-diagnostic, blood work was ordered, and she was admitted.

The admission process seemed an eternity. She signed a boatload of papers, which she carefully read in spite of being rushed. She wondered who was overseeing this harried and hurried ER doctor who so glibly wielded his pen and had her admitted. Her personal odyssey began with a visit to the x-ray department where an angry appearing technician ordered her to stand up and pressed her against a cassette, while she adjusted a number of dials and switches prior to taking the chest x-ray. She was so tired. She was eventually wheeled into her room, which she shared with an elderly woman, who at first glance did not appear to be breathing. This frightening moment passed when the lady started to snore; now fear was displaced by annoyance.

The following morning a cardiologist greeted her at the foot of her bed. His introduction was perfunctory, there was no handshake offered, he did not touch her. He leaned against a wall and began the conversation asking her what had happened. There was so much she wanted to say, how she felt at the moment, her fears, frustrations, and uncertainty. A staccato of questions followed, which only required her to answer yes or no, much as she had learned to do as a trial lawyer, but somehow inappropriate in this situation, not what she expected from a doctor. Within a short period of time he had scribbled a number of orders in her chart, informed her that he was concerned about a possible heart attack, or perhaps a tear in her aorta, or maybe just a gall bladder attack. She wanted to tell him more, about her stress, her father's history of heart disease, and her weight lifting. But then he was gone. There was just the rustling of papers and the swoosh of air as he bolted out of her room. She was alone, terrified, sharing this space with an elderly, somnolent woman, wishing that she had never come. But, the pain had been real and she needed to know.

She was back on the conveyer belt the next morning. She was pushed in a wheelchair to the lab, then to the x-ray department, to the EKG room, back to x-ray. She related that at each stop she felt as if she was dealing with android- like technicians, devoid of any discernable human characteristics, none of whom actually looked into her eyes, engaged her in conversation, asked her how she felt, or touched her. It was as if all this technology was operating independent of human touch, by robots, or some unseen force. Her body parts were figuratively taken apart, studied, recorded, leaving her to feel fragmented and disjointed. She had been given some intravenous medication that made it difficult to think or speak coherently. She had a bedside commode but it took forever for someone to respond when she needed to use it. Her chest pain was now gone but in general she felt worse.

The cardiologist returned the next morning to tell her that she did not have heart disease. For just a moment she had the feeling that he was waiting for her to jump up and give him a hug. Or, was he disappointed that there no more tests he could justify? She asked him about her lungs, aorta, and gall bladder. His answer was patronizing, but reassuring—no problems. And, that was it. Before she could get her clothes on the orderly was in her room with a wheelchair to discharge her. She could not remember if the doctor wanted to see her again.

But, the pains continued. She tried to ignore them. Regular exercise was something she had taken up to relieve her stress, her marital misgivings, her challenge to succeed, and her loneliness. She felt short-changed about her symptoms, she wanted to speak up about her weight lifting, she insisted that there was no opportunity or no invitation to speak. Self discovery provided her with what she needed to know. She eventually realized that overly aggressive weight lifting was the cause of her chest pain. She had come to tell me that she was fed up with our hospital, with our doctors, with the callous and impersonal treatment she received. It wasn't about the cost; her insurance company took care of that. She was simply never going to set foot in our hospital again.

I sat very still throughout this diatribe, transfixed as it were; feeling less and less secure; unable to say anything that remotely referenced coherent thought. It occurred to me that her sojourn through our technologically competent hospital was more a part of the problem, rather than the solution. I was left with the impression that we physicians were unwilling or unable to take the meaning of pain as seriously as we undertook to study its biology. Her journey to Hades began with a hasty and superficial order, a brief moment when her initial doctor scribbled out the order to admit, which led to other such moments with other doctors, whose stake in the process seemed to me more directed at massaging their own focus, rather that focusing on Denise Williams.

We physicians have so much discretionary power with our pens. Other than peer review, where other physicians review the work of a colleague, or in response to a complaint, or an untoward outcome, there is no oversight for order writing. Nor should there be if the physician's motives are honest and focused. Patients simply trust that their well-being is chief amongst the motivations that move physicians, that they carefully write orders that convey quality and concern. Patients are asked to take a leap of faith that the physician has the knowledge, competence, experience, and training to order a test, a procedure or drug that, if used improperly, can cause great harm. Unfortunately, in my experience this is often not the case, that expediency often trumps careful thinking, and the lure of a possible procedure dominates the technophysician's thinking.

A story illustrates this point. Several years ago I was sent a patient who was doing poorly. Another gastroenterologist had previously made the diagnosis of Crohn's Disease, an inflammatory disease of the bowel. The patient had undergone the usual xray and endoscopic studies, including biopsies of the terminal ileum, which is the end of the small bowel and the area where the inflammation was localized. However, cultures of the biopsy material and serologic tests searching for an infection were not done. This is actually not so unusual since Crohn's disease is much more common than other diagnostic possibilities such as tuberculosis, lymphoma or amebiasis. However, the thorough and thoughtful physician would at least consider these less likely possibilities. If the physicians' motive is something other than quality, a hasty approach, which bets on the most likely diagnosis, saves this physician time so that he can move on. In this case the clinical presentation and the radiographs certainly looked like Crohns. The patient was placed on corticosteroids, a reasonable choice if this were Crohn's, but the patient did poorly with persistent weight loss and diarrhea. The patient changed his insurance coverage and ended up in the group where I then practiced. He was initially seen by a family practitioner, a good and conscientious doctor, who continued the orders of the first gastroenterologist. The general practitioner was concerned about the medication that had been ordered, because the patient was doing so poorly; but he was reluctant to change the orders for fear of insulting the gastroenterologist. The family doctor referred him to me, which was a way out of his dilemma since I was now his group's gastroenterologist.

I went over his old records, examined him, and was concerned about his failure to respond. Additional imaging studies were ordered, which revealed a mass in the lower right abdomen. I obtained surgical consultation. He was hospitalized and operated upon. He was found to have a large inflammatory mass, which actually revealed an infection with the protozoa Entamoeba histolytica, not Crohn's Disease. Unfortunately, he died shortly after surgery.

The general practitioner trusted the diagnosis of Crohn's. He was in a position to change the medication, but was reluctant to do it for fear of being presumptuous. This patient should not have died and would not have if he had been placed on the proper anti-protozoan medication in the first place. By the time he was operated upon, the infection was so wide spread and advanced that he could not tolerate the surgery.

If physicians repeatedly write egregious orders, the hospital staff has invested in the medical executive committee and the chief of staff the statutory power to step in. A physician's privileges can be suspended while awaiting an investigatory process, or he/she can be summarily suspended pending a request for a judicial review process, but this rarely happens. This process is laborious, tedious, and labyrinthine. It moves so slowly that time-lapsed photography might be a requirement to verify that it is moving at all. Physicians have a mountain of protection, due process, and procedures to protect their good name, while they are free to continue writing questionable orders. Physician colleagues are loath to take them to task because of the threat of litigation, loss of friendship, and loss of referrals. We physicians are unwilling to sanction our fellows, to carefully review their work, or to defrock them, risking the exposure of more patients to their unsavory ministrations.

There is something about the process of writing orders that is inherently depersonalizing. The physician sits at a desk, usually in his office or at the nurses' station in the hospital, and writes orders that affect a patient's life in a myriad of ways, dissociated from the patient and often oblivious to the issue of suffering. Extraneous influences such as time-management, interruptions, and haste all get folded into the process. Motives other than service, quality, and stewardship compete with baser inclinations. Isolated from the patient, the physician is liable to assume more control over the situation than is warranted. Health care is a corporate affair. In spite of the prevailing attitude held by many technophyisicians, that patients have little to offer or contribute to the process of clinical judgment, there is an overriding obligation to develop a more intimate relationship when making decisions about their affliction and its treatment. Patients are a valuable resource when searching for clinical efficacy, not to be discounted, rather, respected, included, and part of the process. The great clinician, Sir William Osler, has written that the right diagnosis is uncovered within the patient's history 80% of the time. Carefully listening requires a commitment to healing.

Several years ago I visited a hospital in San Diego with a group of medical staff leaders ostensibly to learn about computerized electronic charting. It was an interesting experience. The computer terminals were inside the patient's room. The physician studied that day's lab data, adjusted his therapeutic plan, and wrote his progress note in the patient's room, sharing this event with the patient. There was no opportunity to rehearse or to sanitize the moment; the patient was given the opportunity to share in this activity with the physician, to share in the physician's unadulterated analysis, data integration, and thought processes. There had been some initial concern by the physicians about doing this, having their covers thrown back as it were, but they found to their amazement that the patients loved the experience and that it contributed to communication and compliance. The process was fundamentally changed, by including the patient in the order writing process, at least where concerns of patient comfort were the issue. Outcomes are closely linked to specific therapeutic choices, but the process of becoming, allowing the patient to play a role in order writing, was at least comforting and enabling.

We proposed this methodology to our medical staff and predictably were treated with some hostility. Our physicians wanted time to prepare and write orders in solitude, with a scripted response when they made rounds and talked with their patients. Behavior is hard to change. Physicians want to look good. This was a situation where the physicians wanted to be trusted by their patients, but they did not trust the patients. My experience in San Diego convinced me that watching physicians deal with their medical problems in the raw was a positive experience for patients, one that invited them to become part of the process, one that must occur if patients are allowed to be change agents, by giving them the opportunity to speak up when it comes to issues of their care.

We patients must become more proactive in demanding that we share in this power. Patients should be invited to ask questions about how drugs work, what are the potential complications, and what alternatives are available. By the same token, patients need to know how the diagnostic tools work, and again, the complications and alternatives There is no question in my mind that physicians are the most appropriate persons to write orders, to devise a strategy to deal with an illness, but patients have a vested interest. There may come a time where the electronic chart is commonplace and a locus where the physician and patient can meet and develop a meaningful partnership. This would be one place where patients could ask questions about the use of hi-technology, expensive drugs, and appropriate acuity. Order writing should not remain a mystery, a stealthy substitution for meaningful dialogue. Patients should become familiar with the elements of the written order when they are hospitalized, given a copy of these orders, and invited to participate. Physicians need to be responsible for the orders they write; able to answer questions about expertise without being offended, and insuring that there skills backup their orders.

Patients come to physicians with complaints, which are a window through which we physicians attempt to make some sense of the problem. Physicians take the patient's history and cull out the chief complaint. The nuances of the chief complaint are amplified and detailed with the narrative of the present illness. It is during this process that physicians create a recasting of illness, where the symptoms are reordered to conform to the biomedical theory of practice, a place where illness is often converted into disease. Healing deals with illness, while curing is preoccupied with disease, a huge translocation and at the heart of the health care crisis. Illnesses include the intangible elements of sorrow, fright, and loneliness, often the result of soulful dislocation. We are not simply a bundle of nerves, blood vessels and viscera, responding to an infectious agent or malignant transformation. We are human beings, with a need for solace and hope, elements that derive from a proper divine-human connection, a power available from this connection, often obviating expensive and dangerous technology. Physicians who carefully listen, are open to dialogue, and understand the nature of this power, would have been helpful for Robert Munoz, Melissa White, Denise Williams and the Crohn's patient. The power of the pen is the medium by which we physicians translate their motivations into fruition. This power has the potential for good and evil, depending upon the physician's focus. To take this power away would lead to more mischief, but I believe that it needs to be shared in a meaningful way, and that patients must demand some involvement.

This is ground zero. This is where our health care system is given life, whether for good or bad. So, if we are looking for the genesis of dysfunction, where unsavory events are born, this is the place. This locus is no more the cause of the health care debacle than Logan Airport was the cause of 9/11. However, the dark shadows gather here, given life by the participants involved with the order writing business, and those participants are the doctor and the patient. We will have more to say about that.

To be fair, the new governmental health care program is appropriately invested in eliminating waste, duplication, and redundancy—all byproducts of sloppy order writing. The new health care laws will ultimately deal with this issue with minimal finesse, draconian cost control, and regulations conjured up by health care engineers whose only mission is to cut costs and say employed. This must not happen. There is a dire need to infuse order writing with vigor, but it must be quality, generated by motivated physicians, physicians who are moved to clean up this mess.

Chapter 3
Mary Little A Glimpse Of Excellence

On the occasion of my medical school graduation the commencement speaker spoke to the need of seeing the patient as something more than a malfunctioning body. We were asked to reflect upon the works of Jan Christiaan Smuts, the great South African biologist, statesman, and military leader, who described a way of viewing life, evolution, and bodily processes as part of a universal whole. Somehow, in someway, Einstein's theory of relativity had paved the way for this conceptual model of atoms, cells, and personality representing evolutionary forms of what Dr. Smuts called holism. All life related to the universal, it was not simply isolated and unconnected, and illness was not simply a bodily perturbation caused by some adverse agent. Rather, it was to be seen within the context of the whole being and, as such, connected to the universal whole.

It goes something like this: Sir William Osler has written that 80% of a diagnosis is made from the patient's history. If the physical exam is normal, we physicians are told to pay close attention to the history. If there is profound weight loss, rectal bleeding, difficulty swallowing, the early onset of amenorrhea, profound shortness of breath, or expectorating purulent sputum, then immediate diagnostic and therapeutic intervention is mandated. This would also be the case if there were a disturbing physical finding. To be sure, the initial task is to rule out a physical affliction such as an occult neoplasm, an infectious disease, or an endocrinopathy like hypothyroidism. When the symptoms are less specific and more general, those more characteristic of chronic disease, such as fatigue, lassitude, anorexia, somnolence, and apathy, then this is often due to soulful dislocation, a separation from that universal power we call God. This requires a change in our thinking. This is an area where physicians need help.

This was a challenge to linear thinking, which was difficult for me to swallow since I had spent the previous four years becoming a disciple of causality, learning how to identify the disease process, isolating the responsible agent, and rendering treatment by interrupting the pathologic chain of events. This commencement address challenged my reductionist, mechanistic, Cartesian view of disease, suggesting that there was no separation of mind and body, that the whole was more than the sum of its parts, that human suffering should be seen within this "holistic" framework. As the time I did not find this helpful information, so I relegated it to some subconscious part of my brain.

At the end of the ceremony we took the Hippocratic Oath. We swore by Apollo, the physician, and the god Aesculapius, that we hold sacred these learnings, that we would offer our best to our patients, avoiding the pitfalls of mischievous and deleterious behavior, declining to give deadly medicine or to produce abortions, to abstain from seducing our patients, to protect the doctor-patient relationship, holding conversations confidential, all at the risk of sacrificing our vocation.

This was pretty heavy stuff. Euthanasia and abortions weren't big issues at the time, so I felt comfortable with that part of the oath. The other stuff seemed fairly straightforward. I hadn't yet run into a patient I felt like seducing. Since I was still pretty much filled with the purity of medicine as an honorable vocation, I wasn't sure what mischievous and deleterious behavior might be. Within a moment I felt transformed. As if taking the oath changed me into something or someone quite different. The sun was hot, perspiration dripped from by brow, and I had a hangover from the previous night, yet a mantle of credibility, authenticity, and mystery now seemed to gently drape my shoulders. And for just a moment, a faint touch of transubstantiation. Feeling a bit more divine, a little less human, with a generous dose of grandiosity, I was now the recipient off an ancient legacy.

We were about to enter the cyclical fray of suffering and death. The patients we would first see were clearly ill, with significant signs and symptoms, lending their care to the reductionist methodology we had learned. Only later, mostly after our formal training programs, would we learn about the large mass of patients with chronic disease. Chronic diseases were not the challenge we were first asked to meet. This would come later, without preparation, and generally felt to be an impediment.

******

East Los Angeles is a sprawling community of small single-family dwellings dotting the gentle hills that merge to the east of the city with the San Gabriel Mountains. The streets are curvilinear, built as appendages off one another-- a response to the urban pressure to build more homes. Most of the homes were put up after the Second World War, and some of the tiny lawns probably haven't been mowed since then. Row upon row of towering palm trees put the stamp of Southern California on this community, heavily Latino as any passerby can hear from the hot-blooded music that drifts from open windows. Even in 1961 the visibility was obscured by the incessant smog that shrouded all it touched, from power lines to the hills themselves. In December and January the Santa Ana winds, blowing from east to west, cleared the valley of pollution and, voila-- there it was-- that beautiful costal expanse that stretches from the mountains to the sea. Richard Henry Dana wrote about this beauty, but of course, *Two Years Before The Mast* was written long before the automobile, which has all but destroyed the happy symmetry that existed between the mountains, the inland costal valleys, the sky, and the sea. Dana, a medical student who became partially blind because of measles, was an astute observer while a member of seafaring crew that sailed around Cape Horn to the west coast of America in search of beaver pelts. The opportunity of becoming a doctor was not available for him, but he made the most of his disability, a legacy for future medical students.

The drone of automobiles is the background music omnipresent in Los Angeles. University of Southern California's medical school lies in the shadow of Los Angeles County General Hospital, surrounded by a gargantuan maze of crisscrossing freeways. The hospital, a concrete monster from the 1930s, was the crucible where countless numbers of new doctors learned their craft, where life and death danced ever so dangerously, and where medical students like myself underwent a metamorphosis from wide eyed onlookers to practitioners of the ancient art. The landscape has changed over the years, reflecting the need to build a newer hospital, as well as edifices designed to nourish the needs of medical scientists, researchers, teachers, and students. Yet, the sinews of 1961 are still recognizable and still standing guard.

Basic science, the physical laws that paved the way for man's success as a species, was center stage for the first two years of medical school. This would be the mortar which was to hold together all of our other clinical experiences. If we were to understand pathophysiology we needed to understand physiology; typical reductionist theory so characteristic of allopathic medicine. These were years devoid of color or texture. An inevitable tedium accompanied this intense period of study. Lectures, laboratory time, exams; a structural sameness with different equations and pathways demanded memorization and understanding. Time has a habit of obscuring and amalgamating memories but not feelings. There were feelings of frustration, dread, exhilaration, apprehension, sorrow, and wonder. Many hours were spent in the lecture hall where we spent time intently listening, methodically taking notes, laughing, sweating, and nibbling munchies.

The two basic science years found us fledgling doctors locked in mortal drama with professors who didn't give a shit that we were overworked, stunted by sensory overload, and caught up in the monotony of lectures, labs and study. In retrospect, it was all very necessary, much like boot camp for the military, or spring training for baseball players. At the same time, however, without knowing it, our innocence would be coming to an abrupt halt.

The huge concrete monster benevolently gazed down on our struggles, not yet ready to accept us, yet its shadow a gentle reminder that this was the direction we were headed. Los Angeles County General Hospital was separated from the medical school by Zonal Street. More than a simple street, this border separated the uninitiated from its innards. If we were adequately fortified with the nuances of basic science we would be ready to cross the barrier and invited to become familiar with the processes of healing and dying. The hospital was not interested in diffidence; its expectation was that those of us who crossed would be bold. I struggled with some way to personalize this formidable inanimate object. At once succoring and demanding, I came to call the hospital Mother. It was so near yet so far away. Here was a repository of pathos, a treasure trove of clinical experience, an alchemist's playground where research was converted into clinical tools. So foreboding, Mother watching our every move, arms outstretched inviting us into an intimate experience, yet wary of our insecurities.

When that day came, after that two-year basic science juggernaut, we put on our white coats, straightened them, fastened the buttons, and strode across Zonal Street. This gleaming white monstrosity that served the endless stream of sick and injured East Los Angeles residents, this thing that I now called Mother, was the next stop of our scripted journey. The "yellow brick road" led past a parking structure, up several flights of imposing white steps, and into the inner sanctum. The floor, walls, and ceiling were covered with some type of dull marble, stained with the years of the health care drama, echoing our footsteps and voices, merging them with the background cacophony created by people of all shapes, sizes, and color; a city of 10,000 souls, half of whom were sick, and the other half trying to help. The sights, sounds, and smells were overwhelming, demanding some sort of morbid veneration, an ode to the huge armies of suffering who had traveled these foreboding halls over the years in desperate search of relief. Mother seemed to accept us, but without rank, without much credibility, and with much suspicion. We tentatively approached the elevators. The hospital had 18 floors and very few elevators.

The elevator seemed to have a life of its own. It sliced through the floors, a vertical leap through the layers of the hospital, discharging the sick, the curious, the healers, the teachers, all with a defined role to play in the drama. The hospital was designed like the letter H. The various wards were configured within this architectural rendering. Each wing had a life of its own. The admitting area was close to the elevator, which at times served as a conveyer belt resettling newly arrived patients. The center of each wing was defined by the ward clerk's area. The ward clerk's station was elevated with stools around the outside, like a bar with three sides, where medical students and physicians-in-training could sit and write their reports, where we were introduced to the power of the pen. The ward clerk's station was made of marble--sturdy, indelible, imposing. Sound seemed to bounce off the station adding to the symphony --buzzers, bells, telephones, pagers, elevator doors opening, and gurneys rolling down the tile floors. The ward clerk's station had its own life, a pulsating switchboard where information was received, recorded, transmitted, and where the healers and the sick negotiated their first relationship. The ward clerk was the center of this universe, sitting behind the bar, surrounded by the three monstrous marble counters, managing, facilitating, redirecting; life's representative to this high theater.

The ward clerk who would touch me deeply, who would become part of my life and journey, was Mrs. Lincoln. Lincoln supervised from within the confines of this small bunker, the three arms of which separated her from the rest of mankind, protected, insulated, yet able to reach into the interstices of 7200, an admitting area, with voice, inflection, visage, and will. She occasionally lifted her not inconsiderable self up to waddle here or there, putting her personal stamp on an event, obtaining or transmitting information in a more intimate manner, or sometimes, just visiting. She was strict, respectful, loving, and assertive. There was so much to learn from Lincoln. Countless numbers of young doctors learned from her. Her wisdom both comforted and unnerved many medical students and interns. A large black woman, her voice bounded from the ward clerk's desk, filling every room, every crevice, and every hall way. It was a rather deep voice, sonorous, filled with the melodic rhythm of black America, with a touch of urgency, yet made authentic by its softness. The urgency in Lincoln's voice gave new meaning to the concept of the speed of sound.

Now clinical clerks and nearly indistinguishable from real doctors, we tentatively entered the cyclical fray of life and death. Rotating through the various divisions of the hospital--internal medicine, pediatrics, obstetrics, general surgery--we were assigned patients, required to record their histories properly, examine them and then to present their cases to a member of the faculty. Oral presentations are the way physicians communicate with one another. How one organizes one's thoughts about a patient's chief complaint and how this and other findings are relayed to a peer are time-honored skills to be learned well. Our patients hardly knew we were greenhorns, but to the ward clerks, nurses and faculty our struggles were plain. Having juggled the requirements of each assignment, we were to make our presentation to our faculty advisor in a room just off the wards.

As fate would have it my assignment and faculty advisor would be on Ward 7200, Lincoln's realm. It wasn't long before I began the process of baptism. I was assigned an elderly black female hospitalized with a stroke. The act of assignation was sterile and faceless. A bland piece of paper was handed to me by the chief resident, which listed my name, Hansen, across from my patient, Mary Little. For a few moments I just stood, motionless, carefully studying this piece of paper, as if some intrinsic and profound meaning would somehow leap from the page and sanctify this moment. I was acutely aware that my task was to approach Lincoln who would hopefully direct me to my patient. Lincoln held the keys to the kingdom, the road map, which promised to lead me to Ms. Little, and beyond that, Nirvana. As always, Lincoln was totally engaged, a choreographer of sorts, supervising simultaneous health care dramas, much as an air traffic controller would handle the incessant traffic of flight. She created order out of chaos, part traffic cop, and part switchboard operator, her booming voice a point of reference for both the healers and the afflicted. My task was to get her attention, but not upset the delicate balance that she created, and find the path to Mary Little. Lincoln's eyes were dark, a bit exophthalmic, sending and receiving subliminal messages, always focused. Standing at the throne, a supplicant in spite of my white coat, Lincoln suddenly turned her massive head towards me and focused on my name tag. All of her energy was harnessed and directed for an interminable period of time on my name tag. Why my name tag? After what seemed like an eternity she said, "So, *Mister* Hansen." I think there was more to her opening remarks but at that moment I stood naked before the world. Now everyone within earshot, perhaps all of those involved with health care at Los Angeles County General Hospital, knew that I wasn't actually a doctor. I have this vision of everyone near the throne stopping dead in their tracks, processing the information to which they were all privy. In my dreams I see a multiplicity of eye balls fixed on my name tag, eyeballs that transmitted this information to various parts of their attached brains, allowing for interpretation, preparing for some type of voluntary action which might destroy my ego.

Lincoln's next words were, "bed eight." Her massive head swung to the left, facing one of the women's wards, and with her hand, at once a wand, she pointed out the path. Within a millisecond she returned to other matters which by now were clear to me as being much more important. Gathering my wits as best as possible, visibly sweating, I started on the pathway, walking around all of those eyeballs and brains, which were processing this newly discovered information and which were housed in bodies frozen in space. With fear and trepidation I tentatively gathered my notebook, and examining equipment, and set out on my odyssey.

Deep in the corner of the ward, filled with women engaged in their struggles with illness, I saw the sign Bed 8. A small dark creature was curled up on her side, facing the wall, still as a mouse. As I walked toward the bed I was acutely aware that none of the other twelve patients looked at me, sympathized with me, or acknowledged me. They seemed oblivious to this sentinel event, as if I didn't matter, challenging my ego with relevance. Each was involved with her own affliction, desperately trying to hold off the grim reaper. As if their assignments were more important than mine; as if their indifference to my assignment was appropriate.

Mary Little's bed, like all of the beds in Los Angeles County General Hospital, was a small fortress. The beds were metal, parallel steel bars surrounded Mary Little, which now seemed to be protecting her body from the other patients, from the army of health care persons, from medical students, perhaps, from her own soul. Yet, there seemed to be a soul, perhaps liberated, inviting intimacy, but too ethereal for me to grasp. Mary Little's soul was there, but awaiting my sojourn through the fortress, through the artificial impediment placed by modern medicine to protect her, but at the same time hindering the efforts of those who might want to engage her essence. Her IV bottle was suspended by a prehistoric bird-like contraption, which clanged whenever her bed was touched. No doubt a signal that someone was getting too close. Covers were up to her small head; her hair in tight curls with colored bows; her skin drawn and desiccated; her breathing slow and measured. I introduced myself. There was no answer, no movement. I tentatively touched her head. The prehistoric bird clanged. She moved her head towards mine, our eyes engaged, we sought common ground to define this moment. I introduced myself again, but by now I was aware that she was studying my damn nametag. With a dry mouth, a barely audible, cracking voice, I preempted the situation and introduced my self, *Mister* Hansen, the medical student. Those words tore through the thin veneer of approval I had constructed for myself, handing away my trump card, bearing my own soul to the moment. Conversation was given birth, but slow to develop, two languages searching for meaning.

I had spent nearly two hours examining Mary Little when the resident-in-charge informed me I was killing her. That, of course, pissed me off. The task I needed to learn was how to efficiently extract from Mary Little pertinent information, which would help make a diagnosis and construct a plan of action. The trick was to move things along, to ask questions that obviated the need to communicate in a meaningful way. Part of the perceived success in this training program, from internship through fellowship, was to truncate what the patient had to say. Listening was important, but allowing the patient to tell the story without interruption was not felt to be helpful. I was learning some of what I later had to unlearn. Caught in a dilemma of needing to understand her, but learning to manage my time, I felt an unnatural tension between her need to express herself and my need to get through as fast as possible.

I had learned that the problem was kidney failure. Although I didn't appreciate the resident's attitude, he was helpful by directing me to her major problem at that time, namely the renal insufficiency, not the stroke. What were the possible causes? Which of her medications her kidneys were excreting? Which of these would need to be adjusted? How should we treat her renal failure? What was the relationship between the kidney failure and the stroke?

I was standing with this asshole resident, a cocky blond-haired guy with a toothpick in his mouth and a copy of the New England Journal of Medicine stuffed in his back pocket, when Dr. Fontaine, my professor, suddenly appeared at the patient's bedside, not at the side room where we were to present our assignment, but at the *bedside*. A light-skinned African-American raised and trained in New Orleans, Dr. Fontaine carefully introduced himself to Mary, shook her tiny hand, and with compassion and patience took her history. He let her respond to his questions without interruption, something that I had not learned to do, he nodded understandingly, watching her eyes, maintaining poise and a friendly continence. He carefully examined her, determined to protect her dignity, all the while focused. He pulled out his pencil and calculated on her bed sheets the incremental rise in her blood-urea nitrogen based on her size, dietary intake and present status. A bit taken aback by his casual choice of note pad, I was nonetheless struck by his fund of knowledge and the speed with which he took control. And all the while, in his beautiful, melodic accent, he established and maintained a rapport with this elderly woman, steeping those few minutes in an essence I would later come to recognize as the sanctity of the doctor-patient relationship. I watched and listened, transfixed. He pulled the whole thing off so simply, with dignity, with the poetic, graceful style of a pro. His eyes fixed on hers. He was seemingly oblivious to our presence. Their gazes locked, an undeniable energy seemed to be passing between them. He touched her, caressed her forehead, and engaged her with the elements of healing. Authenticity flowed from his stature and his command of renal esoterica. Both the resident and I stood in awe.

That moment is forever locked in my mind and soul. It has remained as a reminder of what health care is all about. In spite of the vicissitudes that lay ahead, it served as a reference point, an indelible benchmark. My professor and Mary Little were locked in a drama, oblivious of the outside world, sharing an energy that seemed universal, born of the cosmos, defining in a moment a contract for healing. There were no platitudes, no false promises, and no misunderstandings. Their eyes locked, their essences seemed to merge. It didn't take long. Dr. Fontaine's invitation for meaningful rapport was accepted. Healing began right then and there. The renal failure, of course, would respond to medications and dialysis. But the helplessness, the fear, the loneliness, and the insecurity were parts of this affliction that are so common, and remain, in spite of high technology, as a negative force, one that requires healing, not curing. This sentinel moment has been folded within the latticework of these early years. The value of recollection is to sharpen the focus of the present, to hold on to some ballast, endeavoring to unravel the complexities of the contemporary scene. I thank Mary Little and Dr. Fontaine for that moment.

I have come to believe that the magic and mystery of this ideal moment only happens when the industry orchestrates those elements that pave the way for such a meaningful engagement. It can certainly happen independent of our complicated health care system, but it would be a random event, independent of medicine's mandate and mission. This is not necessarily a bad thing, but a better outcome would be a health care system where the elements of the Fontaine-Little encounter are nourished, encouraged, and ultimately commonplace behavior at the point of service

The medical school experience was the bedrock from which ultimately springs understanding and comprehension. Yet, those four years were ephemeral. Within an instant we had graduated. Our heads were filled with facts and book knowledge, but at that moment with so little experience and wisdom.

****

My friend and classmate, Dan Evans, and I set out together to drive to Mazatlan for a much-deserved week's vacation. To be thought of as a doctor brought an instant high. We could now write "M.D." after our names. Traveling the narrow, unadorned highway through Mexican farmland and villages, we reviewed our past four years and examined the future.

"Do you know what you're going to do after your internship?" Evans asked.

I really hadn't thought much about that. The monumental amount of study seemed to have eclipsed any view of what was ahead. I was mostly happy to be through with this phase, being vaguely aware that there were still a number of years of training left before I was a "real doctor." "A residency in internal medicine seems most likely, but I'm not sure after that", I answered.

"Well you'd better start thinking about it," he shot back. Dan was a doer and was always calculating and analyzing.

Somewhat timidly I asked, "Thinking about what?"

Dan fired back, "sub-specialty." He swerved around a group of farmers walking home in the fast-descending darkness. We had driven several hours and intended to keep going until we reached our destination. Then we would renew and have the fun we planned.

"Sub-specialty?" I repeated.

Evans snorted. "There's no money in being another internist, even if you're a good one."

"What do you mean?" I finally asked. I watched a hodgepodge of shanties pass us by, barely visible in the twilight. Small and shack like, they were part of a random world, unaffected by the planning and design which my life knew so well. The world outside this window was amorphous—earthy, primordial, unadulterated. Mine was about right angles, precision, parallel lines. Where did I fit? And here was Evans, spouting as though he knew something I should have picked up on. His attitude irked me.

"It's about gimmicks, Hansen. The future is all about gimmicks. You have to be master of something—the best that's around—to make it now. Medicine is changing. Every smart resident I know is planning to spend another couple of years becoming an expert in some specialty—some nook, some cranny. It's what we're all going have to do. I'm not kidding you, Hansen. You should think about it."

I was silent. He drove hard now, as though to make his point. The car dove around bends in the road like a knife slicing through butter. Evans broke the silence by adding, " Hansen, I believe that there are two truisms you need to keep in mind: The first is that 95% of all patients get well no matter what we do to them. Sure, we are better at treating stuff, but many of these patients would survive whatever we did. Human beings are fantastically resilient. The second is that at the end of life everyone wants you to do whatever to keep the dying person alive. This is an invitation, a carte blanche." These two "truisms" was where Evans believed that gimmicks and sub-specialty came in.

The countryside was swallowed into a quilt of darkness as we pressed onward. I had nothing to say, nothing to offer, but there was lots of time to think.

We spent a week of renewal in Mexico. The beaches were spectacular, white sand appointed like frosting on a cake, gentle aqua-colored waves teasing the sand with harmonic subtleness. We dug our feet into the cool sand and watched the intimate drama of the sea and earth, an embrace, a song of creation, playing those roles, which were played so well many years ago. This beautiful sea, where life took form, its skirt sweeping across the earth's beachhead, a dance of fecundity. The air was humid and teeming with insects. Mexico beckoned us to loose ourselves in its Dionysian amalgam, its sensuous calm, and its ethereal oneness.

This is where it happened for me. This is where I first made a Faustian contract of sorts, willing to exploit the two putative truisms offered by Evans. The frustration of being a good general internist had already occurred to me. I had been looking for a focus, where the depth of disease was more pertinent and the breadth of disease marginalized. This is where the saga of Mary Little began to fade from memory. I'm not sure what goes on in the mind of other physicians who made the decision to enter the cathedral of high technology but I'll bet that the financial payoff played a role, and with time this attitude has a way of adulterating quality, with a free fall into the oblivion of self-service. There was no spiritual ballast to prevent, attenuate, or modify this rush to technomedicine. This vacation left me a bit disturbed, but convinced that Evans was right. We returned to Los Angeles invigorated and nervously anticipating the next several years of training, learning to be specialists, learning the nuances of high technology.

The road to technical competency demands major shifts, translocations, and adjustments as we fledgling specialists climb onto the learning curve. How all this plays out leads to a major impact on the health care crisis. We return to the process of becoming.

Chapter 4
Black Pete: Death Gives Birth To Wisdom

No sooner had we returned from Mexico than we were thrown into the fire, cannon fodder for the sick and suffering. Our uniforms were white smocks and white pants, with large front pockets for stethoscopes, reflex hammers, and notebooks where we kept track of our patients. The very nature of our uniforms invited conformity, which is the bedrock of medical education. July 1st was the opening salvo. I could only stand on the floor where I was assigned and wonder what was going to happen to me and the poor souls I would try to help. For the first half of the century it was commonplace for new graduates to simply hang up their shingle, perhaps learn about doctoring from an older partner, and set sail. It is amazing to me how they could pull that off. In spite of spending several years learning how to be a doctor, I never felt like I was either ready or competent. Technically an MD, with the blessing of the state and organized medicine, I didn't much feel like one. Especially on that first day, which felt like being in a food blender, whirling, noisy, the players in this health care drama going around and around, melting into one another, faceless, impersonal, struggling, an amalgam of humanity with expectations that seemed out of reach. In retrospect, there is no substitution for jumping into the fray, getting one's hands dirty, learning to trust ourselves, and a willingness to ask someone who had the answers. But it was a humbling experience to have graduated from medical school, receiving an impressive diploma, bathing in the accolades from family and friends, and basically not knowing shit. But there I was, feeling much as I had on my first day of medical school, waiting for the first sick patient to swoon into my arms. And, what was I supposed to do?

Before I could take a deep breath and try to make sense out of this scene, Louise Stone headed my way, her face a study of indifference, conserving facial energy by neither smiling nor frowning. I still had visions of Mexico filling my consciousness. I wasn't ready for all of this. Louise had just finished her internship year and she was now my assigned resident. A woman! Put there, no doubt, to test my resolve, my commitment! She was taller than me, her hair cut short, devoid of makeup, her voice forceful and gravely. She smelled strongly of tobacco and on that first day she shook my hand and announced, "My name is Dr. Stone." At that moment she became horseface to me. She did have a long equine visage, a cartoon character of sort, but since she was officially my boss, I needed to clean up my act. My list of tasks, affectionately called scut work, was tremendous that first morning. I had made the mistake of asking Horseface what she would like me to do. As if it wasn't obvious. She had admitted some 30 patients within the previous 24 hours and she needed help. You could palpate the tension in the air.

Starting the third IV of the morning became a major challenge given the discovery that there weren't any more needles in my little area. Panic began to rear its ugly head. There were two more IVs to start and a ward of 15 patients quietly watching every move. Horseface chose to poke her head in, a not so subtle reminder that procedures still needed to be done, most of the patients didn't have histories and physical exams, and daily rounds would begin in 20 minutes. To the 15 patients who watched , it was clear that there was an organizational melt down. Horseface couldn't care less.

Now after one week OJT, we were asked to present a case to Black Pete, a most feared faculty person, the faculty person that could melt steel with his eyes, not so much a person, but an frightening experience, dressed up like a faculty person, well known to generations of USC medical students, and the faculty person scheduled to descend upon us this day. This felt like the first time in a varsity game, perhaps the way soldiers feel with their first combat experience. "All right you goats, lets go", Maddox barked. Phil Maddox was the chief medical resident on our floor. Maddox must have weighed more than 300 pounds, disheveled, sweating, a high squeaky voice, a face scared from teenage ache, but smart! Christ, was he smart! The chief resident was a fourth year medical resident, usually at the top of the resident class, someone who chose to do an additional year in internal medicine, often a fat person. He had been through it all, had seen it all, learned to manage his time without killing too many patients and without pissing off too many attending physicians, and he was our chief resident. The chief resident presides over daily rounds, which included several residents and their interns from a particular service. Ours was internal medicine and we were housed on the 7th floor, near 7200 where Lincoln prowled. Rounds usually started in the ICU because those were the patients who needed the most help, where we physicians-in-training needed the most help. We were affectionately called goats, although we more like sheep, following our leaders, never complaining out loud, never questioning what we were told, information lifted from the weighty volumes of medical science, which had accumulated over the years. Maddox also seemed to sense danger in the air as he had many encounters with Black Pete during his four years. He informed us that he did not need any more of this shit, since he would be finished with his training at the end of the year

Horseface gathered the charts together. The charts had metal covers and were piled on top of each other in a pushcart that looked like a grocery cart. Lucky me was given the task of pushing the grocery cart. The thing squeaked, listing to one side, and threatened to turn into a catastrophe. Charts were piled too high and kept sliding off onto the floor, and when an individual patient's bed was reached it was my job to fumble through the mass of metal and produce the appropriate chart. I knew very little about these patients, which was very understandable to me, but not to Maddox, our chief medical resident, and certainly not to Horseface, whose organizational skills and medical acumen would be shredded if these cases weren't down pat. Wisdom would eventually lend a hand in managing all of that, but inexperience held center court.

Black Pete was bigger than life. He had taught several classes during our medical school experience, so many of the trainees, who had graduated from USC, had been exposed to his celebrity.. Everyone from the voluntary faculty, to the chief resident, to Horseface, to the interns, and to the lowly medical students were nervous and fidgeting. This was the kind of event that could make or break a career. But one of us was missing. Our group, which was composed of Horseface, Maddux, myself, and Gordon Rather was not complete. Time was flying and I could see Black Pete in my mind shifting from one foot to another, surrounded by the visiting faculty, nurses, ancillary personnel, and administrators. Where the hell was Rather. Horseface began to turn on me, as if I was responsible for him, but maybe I was. Maybe that was something else I needed to learn.

July often brings insufferable heat to Los Angeles. Los Angeles

James T. Hansen, M.D.

County Hospital was built in the 30s and had few amenities, especially air conditioning. The smog was so bad on certain days that the view within the hospital was fuzzy, indistinct, and intimidating. As fate would have it, Gordon Rather and I were assigned to Horseface's internal medicine rotation. Rotating internships were the norm in 1965. Interns spent each month in a different venue, helping us decide which career path to choose. Most of us were pretty certain about this, but we were expected to have a well-rounded learning experience. Today, young doctors are more focused from the get-go since the process of becoming a specialist is so lengthy,

at times being a six to seven year process for the most demanding specialties. In an effort to truncate the arduous process young doctors dive right into their specialty of choice and offered a path that eliminates the internship year. Although I understand the reasons for this accelerated pathway, what is lost is the breadth of experience and a familiarity with a wider range of illness provided by a general internship.

Gordon Rather was a singularly interesting person. Born and raised on the east coast, Ivy League educated, meticulous, patient, confident of himself, he was a work of art. We developed a friendship in medical school, which has lasted all of our lives. Rather had that especial characteristic of grace under pressure. He never seemed to be rattled, he often chided me for being uptight, and he seamlessly blended levity, focus, and patience. As our little team walked nervously down the hallway, we peeked in each of the patient rooms frantically searching for Rather, whose absence might ignite Black Pete.

When all seemed to be lost, we found him, in a male ward. Rather, who was a stickler for completeness, had just about finished a physical exam on a very thin, unkempt, and malodorous man, whose admitting diagnosis was rectal bleeding. An integral part of the physical exam, especially with this type of case, would be a rectal exam. The large patient holding rooms were separated according to sex and severity. This particular patient, one that we often referred to as a GOMER, (i.e. get out of my emergency room) was not in the least bit interested in having a rectal exam done on him. By the same token, Rather was not interested in signing off on an incomplete physical exam. When we stuck our heads into the ward where the two of them were, we stopped in our tracks. There was the patient, clothed only in an upper torso gown, with the backside open, on his hands and knees scurrying away from Rather. But, right behind him, also on his hands and knees, was Rather, his right hand gloved with lubricant on the index finger, scurrying right behind the patient, feinting with his gloved finger toward the man's anal opening, but falling short when the man scurried faster with a burst of energy, his manhood flapping in the breeze. Rather was composed, unflappable, focused, and hell bent on getting this job done. His tie was stuffed into his shirt and his shirtsleeves were rolled up anticipating the worst. Patients on the ward, many of whom were on death's doorstep, raised themselves up, choosing to either urge Rather on, or to side with the scurrying patient. It became a fierce contest. The combatants were cheered on; only in this case the cheerleaders were frail, cadaveric, morose men who had found a moment of respite provided by the encounter.

Rather finally cornered the guy and thrust his lubricated index finger into the delicate orifice, while our disheveled patient bellowed, whined, threatened and cajoled. The marriage of dedicated intent and abject avoidance created a surreal theater, thoroughly entertaining the representatives of misery and suffering, and, for just a moment, laughter trumped doom, rekindling hope, and put the grim reaper in retreat. Laughter was a rare commodity on admitting days, but this brief respite not only provided levity, but has lasted a life-time in my memory. While it says a lot about human nature, the value of levity in healing, and the dignity of man, it goes to the heart of behavior instilled into medical students and house officer during the process of becoming a doctor.

We are taught to be meticulous in history taking and doing a physical exam. There are lectures, reading material, and demonstrations to guide us with these myriad facets of doctoring. The reasons we do it this way are multiple: to get a good grade, to learn how a good doctor does it, to pander to our obsessive nature, to enhance our resumes in preparation for becoming an active staff member in a hospital, or because that is the way it has always been. Like most of us, Rather was driven by the need to be in possession of those tools which would define who he was, which would pave the way for him to become a member of the fraternity of doctors who are members of the active medical staffs of the better hospitals, who are insured of a successful career. We are taught to emulate our teachers, do it the way we are shown, and woe be it to the fledgling doctor who disdains this advice, since the issue of getting a good residency was at stake. Residencies were where we learned to do the procedures or surgeries, and the gimmicks which would ultimately define who we were. So much is at stake. Having gathered Rather up, wet with perspiration, out of breath, and basking in the glow of a successful rectal exam, we moved toward our encounter with Black Pete. Horseface and Maddox stood by incredulously with their mouths gaping open during this event.

The script for grand rounds is well choreographed, having been honed by myriads of interns, residents, and faculty over the years. A particular case was usually presented by the resident, with the chief resident nervously standing by, and the intern simply a *gofer*, someone who retrieved needed data from the chart when asked by the resident, someone whose job it was to learn, to translate what we had been taught in the classroom into meaningful doctoring, so that we could move up the sides of the pyramid, and ultimately become "real" doctors. Those who could not handle the task, who could not make it to the top of the pyramid, simply fell asunder, finding another venue for continuing the process. Medical students compete for the better internships and fellowships predicated on their academic standing and in-house performance. Faculty made rounds on a weekly basis, or more often when needed, reviewing the most interesting and demanding cases during the week. This was a nerve wracking event, testing the mettle of the entire pecking order of the fledgling health care team, and certainly not the kind of thing expected on the first week as an intern. But, there it was. Black Pete was the prototypical faculty person. Tall and athletic, blessed with a stentorian voice, he was bigger than life. When he strode with those long, lanky legs onto a stage or to a patient's bedside, a quiet ruffling of the air filled the room and bathed us all with his largesse. Black Pete's name came from his thick, black hair, which outlined his chiseled visage in a way that invited total attention. He was a full professor of medicine with a focus on liver disease. But he seemed to know everything. His teaching method was more at home on a football practice field. His piercing dark eyes locked on to whatever poor soul was trying to answer his question. His intensity framed the edges of the moment in a way that converted a learning opportunity into an indelible experience. He wasn't someone striving for higher ground in order to define his persona. He *was* hepatology, he *was* medicine, a seasoned veteran, the author of a plethora of articles and text books. His reputation preceded him wherever he went and most especially with every new class of fledgling doctors. More than one student or trainee buckled under the intensity of his gaze while Black Pete awaited the correct answer. He could accept a wrong answer, because that gave him an opportunity to teach, but woe be it to the unlucky person who tried to bullshit him. He could reduce the pomposity and self righteous behavior of a smart ass to an amorphous mass of gelatinous slither. His lessons were never forgotten, especially on those occasions when egos were shred and reduced to dust.

Mrs. Gentry was a 86 year old white female who had been admitted on my service with pneumonia. She struggled for several days with a high fever, shallow respirations, and a cough productive of purulent sputum. She was one of the patients that had been selected by the chief resident to be presented to Black Pete. She had become less responsive during the preceding days, refusing to eat, and talking about death. That got her transferred to the ICU. She seemed to be giving up, unwilling or unable to expectorate the infected sputum. She resisted being taken to the x-ray department for her daily chest x-ray, she actually tried to fight off the orderlies, but she was too weak to resist. I tried to explain to her that she was to be the subject of a small conference, but she waved me away, she had a vacant and distant look. Initially intelligible, she became vacuous. This was bothersome to me, but Horseface had made it abundantly clear that I needed to triage patients, to manage my time because of the incredible demands, to limit my involvement with any particular patient if the issues were not directly related to the disease. She made it clear that the pertinent information related to the pathophysiology of the disease, the scientific basis for the disease was what was important, and that time spent in this endeavor was well spent in an effort to find a cure.

I was uneasy, sensing that Mrs. Gentry wanted to communicate with me, yet there was not time and that was not my job. She often reached out for my arm, her skeletal fingers grasping my forearm, pulling my head closer to her lips that seemed intent on telling me something. But what did she have to offer that was more important than my physical exam, the laboratory data, and being made ready for presentation at grand rounds?

Black Pete arrived imperiously on our ward. He was accompanied by several private physicians, interns, and residents, all totally mesmerized by his pronouncements, engulfed by his largesse, carefully asking questions avoiding those pitfalls that would lead to that awful moment when he would simply stare at the questioner, his gaze penetrating, his brow furrowed, with a pedantic response that could freeze molten steel. The assembly surrounded Mrs. Gentry's bed. Her nurse rustled around her, straightening her bed clothes, closing the drapes that protected her from curious onlookers. Mrs. Gentry was oblivious to the moment, or at least she seemed to be. Her eyes were closed, there was an air of defiance, or perhaps resignation. Nasal prongs supplied needed oxygen, her IV provided her with needed hydration and a conduit for medications, her catheter creeping out from beneath the bedclothes delivered urine into a bag.

I was asked to present her case. I described why she had come to the hospital, what her complaints were, what our findings were, including the physical exam, the lab work, and her x-rays. I was scared shitless. Hoping not to be asked any questions by Black Pete, I carefully presented the data. Several doctors carefully asked questions, which I answered just as carefully. The stage was now set for Black Pete to flash his brilliance, that magic we all waited for, the moment when we could define ourselves in relation to this giant.

Black Pete spent the first several moments outlining a differential diagnosis based on the data, inviting us to stretch beyond the obvious, challenging us to think outside the box and consider less likely diagnoses. No one said a word. Black Pete's acumen and intelligence had us in his spell. Things were going well. Black Pete seemed satisfied that the patient was being well cared for, no one asked stupid questions. Typically, after the presentation and analysis by Black Pete, the moment would come when he approached the patient to ask her questions, and to verify her history. He approached the head of the bed and grasped her hand. Something was wrong. Anguish was beginning to linger in the air, feet shuffled, and silence was punctuated by whispered voices.

Black Pete turned his head towards me. This was unexpected. I had done my job. It was for others who were further along in the educational process to participate in the discussion. But Black Pete was staring at me, an innocent intern, now with visible sweat on my brow. I detected some very muted giggling amongst my fellow interns, and disdain on the faces of Horseface, Maddux, Rather, and the more seasoned doctors. Black Pete looked at my name tag, reminiscent of Mrs. Lincoln, studied it for a short period of time, and said "Hansen, come over here and tell us what's wrong." My mouth was dry. I was confused. What had gone wrong? Black Pete took her hand and placed it into mine. It was cold, there was no pulse, I now understood, although this revelation was unwanted.

Mrs. Gentry had died during the presentation. I would have been less shaken if thermonuclear war had broken out. Once again the sinews of my being were under attack. What flashed before my eyes, lingering for only moment, was the understanding now that Mrs. Gentry might have been trying to tell me that she was going to die, or wanted to die. But dying was not part of our lexicon. Doctors were there to learn how to save lives, how to cure, how to dismantle the grim reaper.

Black Pete seemed beside himself. I suspect this was the first time such a thing had happened to him. Perhaps out of pity for me, or simply insouciance, he walked away, trailed by the gaggle of doctors who continued to mumble to themselves. Rather playfully slapped me on the shoulder, winked, and let out his breath. Mrs. Gentry's nurse had pity for me, holding my hand and reminding me that we had done what we could. Or had we? In retrospect it is clear to me that a chance for meaningful healing was missed because I could not reach out beyond what I had so meticulously studied. I assumed that all of her distress was simply related to the pneumonia. It never occurred to me that this was a being that needed to communicate about global issues, her fear of dying, was it going to be painful, was there any hope, or did she do something wrong. This is where spirituality would have been helpful; helping her connect to her higher power, not so much a surrender, but subordinating her ego to that benevolent higher power. We were not taught any of this stuff. I was locked into a textbook. Black Pete, along with the other professors who would guide us, grade us, and pass us on, had become more important than any metaphysical ideals that may have been floating around. Our focus was to emulate our teachers, subordinating individual thoughts and ideas to the task at hand.

Up to this point medical school had been a game of sorts. The adventure of learning and the anticipation of patient care obscured the profound realities of what this was all about. Although totally engulfed with the internship year, now *real* doctors, it would take two additional isolated events to crash through the fortress of my naiveté.

Judy Springer was a beautiful young woman admitted as a drug overdose patient one hot July night. She was in coma. A comatose patient presents a number of possibilities as to the cause. It was high theater. Was this a head injury? Meningitis? Stroke? If the patient is a female with bleached-blond hair and finger and toenail polish, although chauvinistic, the conventional wisdom is that "drug overdose" goes right to the top of the differential-diagnosis list. As insensitive as this sounds, this attitude has proven expeditious and lifesaving. Judy Springer was indeed a drug-overdose patient, barely breathing, vital signs fragile, and hypothermic. All of her signs were bad. She was immediately sent to the ICU. Our first task was a dual one: to identify the offending agent and simultaneously sustain her blood pressure and respirations. Judy underwent gastric lavage, an endotracheal tube was inserted, and a central line established to monitor her heart action. She stayed in a coma for nearly two weeks.

Samuel Owens, a quintessential hippie, and I managed most of her basic care. We had no idea who she was, where she came from, what she thought or why she had wound up like this. An older couple visited her infrequently. We thought they were her parents but we weren't sure. They slipped in quietly, stood a silent vigil, and then were gone. On one or two occasions a guy about our age visited. He introduced himself as Randy. His hair was long and scraggly. He wore a wooden cross around his neck, jeans, an open shirt, and sandals. He reminded me a little of Owens. He would talk quietly to her, all the while brushing her brow. But mostly she was alone; eyes closed, very still, a goddess.

Eventually the ENT resident decided to replace Judy's endotracheal tube with a tracheotomy, a breathing tube surgically placed into her windpipe that was the standard course of action for any patient who continues to remain in a coma for a prolonged period of time. The tracheostomy was a safer, a more secure way of maintaining her airway and would keep her well suctioned. The only time Judy moved was when the nurse placed the suctioning device in her tracheotomy. She gagged, coughed and writhed. Judy was beautiful, delicate and enchanting in her quiet repose. Owens and I talked to her whenever we could. Deep down we hoped we could will her to life. We fantasized about the day she would blink open her eyes and offer us her hand. Was she married? Did she have a lover? Owens and I were already in love with her. Her radiance sanitized the range of unpleasant tasks required to keep her clean and healthy: body wastes to be washed away; secretions to be suctioned, bedsores that needed debridement and cleansing, and foul odors from her respirator and nasogastric tube. Not a single one of these obscured her loveliness.

And then it happened. There was no warning. Like the petals of a morning rose unfolding, Judy opened her eyes. They flickered at first, as we had imagined they would, and they stayed open. Azure blue, glazed and filmy for seconds at first, then glistening and clear, fixed on her surroundings, following the movements of people around her, beginning to comprehend.

Before long Judy could whisper words when she was shown how to cover her tracheotomy. She began to eat, sit up and smile. She remained confused, unable to grasp the magnitude of events that had brought her to us, but her smile was real and we were captivated. Owens and I stopped by her bed in the ICU whenever possible, keeping our conversations simple, never pressing her for the answers we so desperately wanted to know, mindful of how fragile she was and how careful we needed to be with her.

Owens would always start by saying "Judy, just checking on how you're doing." It always seemed an insipid way of talking to a princess. She would just smile and make my knees weak. We would take turns asking her if there was someone we could call, if she wanted to write a note, if there was anything else we could do. She would just smile and shake her head no.

There was always a massive amount of work to do. It was still July, oppressive and smoggy, and Owens and I had admitted over two dozen patients during the night. Thank God for amphetamines. By late morning, our heads were ringing and our nerves were frayed. I was beginning a bone-marrow exam on a woman with a low white-cell count two beds down from Judy. The nurse was handing me a syringe filled with anesthetic when I heard Owens' voice through the drawn curtains. "Hansen, come here."

"Hold on." "I need a couple of minutes," I replied.

"Hansen, like now, man," hissed Owens, urgency in his voice.

I handed the syringe back to the nurse and strode through the curtains. Owens stood by Judy's bedside.

The ICU had been filled with eerie stillness. And now this was shattered. A crash cart carrying emergency medicines and equipment was rushed to Judy's curtained bed, a code status was called over the PA, and emergency lights were pulsating. Nurses, respiratory techs and the EKG tech were closing in on Judy. I threw back the drapes.

Rather had his fingers pressed against the bright red blood that spurted from Judy's gurgling tracheotomy wound. Judy, her face frozen with panic, amazement and resignation, was staring straight ahead; her eyes wide open as she grabbed my arm with her right hand.

It was clear that even Judy knew she had a tear in an artery, the fountain of pulsating bright red blood could not be missed. We learned later that this was caused by friction from the tracheotomy appliance against the innominate artery, which lays near the trachea. Oxygenated blood, pulsating from the contractile action of the heart, is a source of wonder, a life giving fluid, but when it sprays into the air it is a messenger of death. Owens agonized in a classic medical-emergency dilemma. Compressing the artery to control the bleeding occluded Judy's airway, suffocating her, but if he allowed her to breathe, blood flooded her airway. The ENT resident could do nothing without immediate surgery. We all stood there, waiting for the resident, unable to do a thing but stare in disbelief as Judy drowned, asphyxiated and bled to death before us within ten minutes.

Owens cried as she let go of my arm and the life went out of her eyes. I did nothing. Perhaps it was machismo, stoicism or the lessons I was finally absorbing from Horseface. I simply could not show a single emotion.

We had been practicing the motions of professionals--putting personal things aside, rising above petty concerns and actively confronting the challenges at hand. Our training was teaching us to substitute denial, play-acting and even self-deception for authentic responses that might slow us down, eat up time, and dilute profits. We were distancing ourselves further from the mystery of the doctor-patient encounter. We had forgotten what Dr. Fontaine showed us. The work we did had its place in a system; to be less than professional would mean obstruction to the smoothness, speed and efficiency of the system. We were deliberately cultivating profound shortcomings.

In the wake of Judy's death I attacked the bottle. I had nowhere to turn. Rage, fear and abandonment boiled deep inside of me, tumbling me back in time to an early stage of my own evolution, where outlines were unclear, events and people murky. I had no notion of how to deal with this. It rumbled in a buried, hidden hollow within me, and as it now began to growl and roll towards the surface. I had nowhere to turn.

So I drank. I drank and I drank and I drank. I attacked the bottle, losing myself in its soothing balm, offering alcohol to the demons that cried inside me for revenge. A Sisyphean effort to quell the fires of rage, insanity and hysteria leaped through my guts. Judy's sweet smile everywhere in my brain, I had a few beers, then some gin, then more gin, and laughing, crying, I passed out. Fortunately I had a couple of days off. I spent the next day in and out of sleep, unable to eat, reliving that awful moment--that grotesque red fountain, the loss, and my anguish. This was the first time that I had seen a person die, the first time I had seen death trump modern medicine, and the first time I had seen a beautiful, young person suddenly become a corpse.

*****

August brought more heat, smog and sick patients. The Grief for Judy had to take a back seat, as there were so many other patients. The scales were tipping, as they never had before. A night came with 25 patients per intern- congestive heart failure, severe pneumonia, strokes, heat exhaustion, bleeding ulcers and cirrhosis. At the end of 36 hours, I was more than grateful to fall into bed. Sleep came in milliseconds. I dreamt of hunting ducks with my father. Beautiful mallards hovered on a lake, there

Reinvent the Heal

for the taking -boom, boom, boom. But this was not a dream: There was somebody pounding on my door. I staggered to open it. A security guard was talking frantically. "Dr. Hansen, there's an emergency. All interns are to report to the MAR."

"What's this, a joke?" I demanded.

"No sir. My orders are I've got to get all you guys up and going."

We had once had a drill like this in medical school. I got myself together, yanking on my clothes, my distinctive white uniform, and as I glanced out of my ten story window, smoke rose in the distance, over South-Central Los Angeles.

The year was 1965. The first US troops had arrived in Viet Nam, Malcolm X was shot to death , the Dodgers would win the World Series, and Winston Churchill passed away. Civil rights was a hot topic. This was the year of the Selma march. Lyndon Johnson was the president. There was a general restlessness and uneasiness within the African-American community in Los Angeles, which mirrored similar feelings in the country at large. Attitudes and perceptions were changing. All of this was occurring while I was totally preoccupied with the job of learning to be a doctor, but reality would soon invade my space.

It was total bedlam in the admitting room. I pieced together that there was some sort of riot going on. Fires raged over the Watts area of Los Angeles. The night air was filled with the wailing of sirens, urgency was palpable, constant movement, conversation was reduced to the essential, orders barked, messages sent and received, police radios blaring.

The admitting room cubicles were filled with young black men, fire fighters, and those who were in the wrong place at the wrong time. Many of the wounds were from gunshots. There were fire fighters with gun shot wounds in their backs. There were several black youths with Achilles tendons cut from bounding through broken store windows as they made off with stolen loot. Others, both black and white, were fatally injured just because they were in the wrong place at the wrong time. The smell of smoke, gunpowder and burned flesh pervaded my senses My olfactory and auditory senses were overloaded. The standard triage system was used. Patients lethally wounded were simply made as comfortable as possible; those with minimal wounds were asked to help those with more serious wounds. Sorting out patients with more serious wounds took precedence. No one had time for casual conversation. Adrenaline flowed, and skills I didn't think I owned soared into action. Venous cut downs, a minor surgical technique of placing a large caliber catheter into a brachial vein, jumped into place, chest tubes fell in effortlessly, simple fractures were quickly set, and superficial lacerations were sutured as if by some other power. Everywhere was the sound of crying, moaning, yelling, swearing, angry words, and beepers filling the air.

For the most part I was focused on what was immediately before me. I was aware of fellow interns near by, but their proximity was felt rather than seen. Sweat poured from my brow. My lips were parched but strangely I was not thirsty. I felt light on my feet. I intuitively sensed a presence. At first it was simply an amorphous figure, not inanimate, but somehow reaching out with anguish. Within an instant it was gone, replaced by a thin haze of what seemed like smoke. There was less clarity; outlines were less distinct, yet this was only a vague feeling. Ambulances followed one another discharging casualties like an assembly line. Police officers were everywhere, authority was subordinated to confusion, weapons at the ready, but unsure what to do. Blood was everywhere.

A sickly stickiness made walking unpleasant. I would lift my eyes from time to time to gather my wits and then I saw a figure, which was no longer an amorphous mass. It was a large black woman with tears in her eyes, her head bowed, engulfed by anguish. Then, she was gone, but I knew it was Lincoln. It didn't matter why she was there; only that she was there, clearly staking out a claim even in this totally dysfunctional human drama. Not a voyeur, not an adversary, not a saint, but joining hands with all of us, the hospital team and the rioters, the police and the looters, accepting all of us, grieving as part of the whole, sharing in a subliminal force and ever ready to pour this force into the mixture. For a brief instant I felt part of a larger totality, bonded with all human beings, a glow that was shattered when the realities of the tasks before me invaded my space.

The Watts riot changed the fragile détente that existed between Los Angeles's African-American community and its white community. Attitudes changed, a residue of hostility permeated our hospital ever so subtly, but unmistakably present. The easy to and fro banter between us white doctors and the black nurses, elevator operators, the housekeepers, and the medical technicians, was displaced by feelings of distrust, hostility, and remorse. It wasn't overly obvious, it was barely palpable, but it was there. The civil rights movement was fully engaged and this dispossessed group was more demanding.

The horror! The horror! Kurtz said it all in Conrad's *Heart of Darkness*. Suffering and absurdity were becoming all too commonplace. The ebb and flow of life was jostled by events such as these allowing a glimpse of chaos that was unsettling in the least. These events stand out and have had a profound affect on my life. For the first time I could see suffering for what it was. It had been so abstract. Now it was in my face. Dealing with the dark side of health care is a challenge for anyone. Death and dying were demanding respect. When death becomes the enemy, the business of doctoring takes on a new face. To lose a patient in spite of giving it our best is an invitation to melancholy. Our definitions of success are intimately tied up with survival, additional life, and victory over disease. The process of healing, of soothing a distraught soul, is often an afterthought. The process of change that is attendant upon any sickness is obfuscated by the need to conquer death. To surrender or give in is seen as ignominious. That is not to say that technomedicine does not have a place where saving a life is possible. It certainly would have been helpful for Judy Springer. Yet, so much of what I have seen cries out for support and strengthening those peculiarly human assets that protect and aid the process of transformation. Dying is part of life, and this phase of life is worthwhile and valuable. Making every effort to reverse what seems reversible is worthwhile. However, sometimes returning the person to wholeness is futile. Sometimes prolonging life is futile. Sometimes changing the course of an inexorable illness is futile. Hope is never futile. Quality medical care, which is often a casualty when left to we technophysicians, has more to do with the value of what is left of life than a presumptuous victory over death.

Grief left its imprint after those years of training. These cases, Evans' admonition, and the four years of training helped make my decision to find a gimmick and choose a specialty, which I believed would give me more control, more protection from the harpies that cried out with death and dying, and free me from being intimate with the horror. For each step I marched towards technical competency, I distanced myself further from the mandate of healing. I was learning how to probe the depths of disease with the tools of modern medicine. Gastroenterology was my choice of specialty, not because I necessarily liked orifices, not because the process of digestion and assimilation were high on my list of trophies, but because this was essentially a new specialty, with new technology, which promised distance between me and suffering, yet a conscious decision that promised financial success and provided stature. The seduction by Evans was complete. Indeed, there were countless numbers of suffering souls, but there was precious little time to identify with patients, to feel their plight, sound out their feelings, assimilate their misery and anoint them with that mythic, fragrant oil of healing. Soon I would be able to gauge illness from afar, minister dispassionately, reach into bodily dysfunction with the miracles of technology and rewire, and reorder all its broken circuitry. Altruism was fading from sight. Whatever idealistic motives that were initially present, the quest to become a technophysician had its way and the purity of healthcare was left adulterated. I was on my way. Fortune smiled ahead of me and somewhere behind, in the dimming recesses of the road, the memory of Lincoln, Black Pete, the saga of Judy, and the Watts riot faded from view. I moved quickly toward my future. The wisdom of my guides, now ghosts, fought for one last glimmer. Then they were gone. But I had one more lesson to learn and it had to do with the pharmaceutical industry, known as Big Pharma. My experience with this industry introduced me to the realities of practicing medicine as well as some early insight into the dysfunction of doctoring.

Chapter 5
Drug Day The Seduction By Big Pharma

Of all the inconsistencies, of all the ironies, and of all the paradoxes of medical education, the one that is most securely fixed in my mind is drug day. The main auditorium of Los Angeles County General Hospital was a spacious room, often the sight of fine arts, lectures, and medical presentations, and as such a treasure for many of the 5000 that worked in this health care arena. The room was on the first floor, with seating room for hundreds, boasting state of the art acoustical and lighting systems and an imposing stage. But, for one hour, on the fourth Thursday of the month, it became a carnival of sorts, a marketplace for physicians ostensibly focused on new pharmaceuticals, called drug day. On the surface that isn't too bad if it was only an educational experience. But, this was capitalism at its worst, within the bosom of a healing, teaching, and research institution, and as such, out of place. Here, on this fourth Thursday, the main auditorium was invaded by pharmaceutical representatives, sent to pitch their wares, new drugs, using their polished marketing skills to new doctors in training. Yet, the attraction was undeniable. Drug day was glitzy, sexy, and seductive. Here, within short reach of the amorphous mass of suffering, dedicated healers, focused teachers, and prime time researchers, was the Barnum and Bailey of health care. We young medical students and physicians understood this paradox on some level, but we were bought and sold just the same. It is not as if we weren't warned about this type of predatory behavior. Many of those professors who were charged with mentoring us attempted to fortify our resolve to remain above the fray, to hold on to professionalism. But, alas!

James T. Hansen, M.D.

John Webber was the chair of the department of pharmacology. He was not an MD, rather a PhD, which was beginning to be the norm for professors teaching basic science in medical schools in the early 1960s. He was tall, patrician in appearance, melodious voice, and a very intense man. He used body language to make a point, redefining manual dexterity, with flourishes of his hands for emphasis. The libretto of his lectures always included an admonition to read the basic science regarding a new drug, to avoid like the plague the ministrations of the pharmaceutical representatives, and to make decisions regarding drugs utilizing study and understanding. This was his passion. He was a benevolent sort of guy, never actually denigrating pharmaceutical company practices, but inviting those of us about to become doctors to use our thinking caps when making choices regarding drugs. Much of this was lost on deaf ears, especially when it came to drug day. I'm not sure why this was so. I suppose a significant number of my medical school colleagues actually looked upon this event as a learning experience, listening closely to the well honed pitches, oblivious to the bestial attraction offered up by beautiful sales reps. Many of us had come to see this experience through cynical eyes. There were the mixed messages we got about doctoring, the attraction of future dollars to be earned, the respite from the tedium of lectures and study, and the rather tenuous hold on the spiritual dimensions of healing

In Dr. Webber's lectures we studied the structure and function of drugs, learned about the applied biochemistry, studied formulas, interactions, metabolism, and reactions. We leaned how drugs were synthesized, distributed in the body, and how they achieved the goal of repairing the afflicted bodily system. We also leaned that many drugs were simply modifications of herbs and plants used for decades by healers and shamans.

As part of Dr. Webber's course we learned that until the 1950s the AMA assumed a watchdog role in investigating and culling out dangerous drugs from meaningless pharmaceuticals. The AMA gave up this vocation, only to have conservative physicians, in powerful AMA positions, sally up to big business, the pharmaceutical companies, and form a détente, which promised the return of profitable drug advertising to the AMA. A gauntlet was thrown to the pharmaceutical companies; they would be given the power to attest to the efficacy and safety of new drugs, leaving out the FDA, if they would return to the AMA fold and provide financial support through magazine advertising. This is the place where Professor Webber steps in. He fully realized the potential persuasive powers of these pharmaceutical companies to seduce and influence physician-ordering practices. Recall, physicians are the only ones with the power of the pen. It wasn't long before beautiful pharmaceutical representatives arrived on the scene, making a pitch for their product, and putting physicians in their back pocket. And, if they were not persuasive enough, there were wonderful gifts and trips to exotic places, which cemented the deal. This was the era where drug advertising was aimed at physicians who had the sole power to order them.

I learned that physician ordering practices reflected these industrial influences, and audits of physician behavior have uncovered this bias and the results of the sales effort, where the marketing and promotional efforts of drug companies eclipse the proper scientific indications for drugs. In other words, for various reasons, physicians were seduced by pharmaceutical companies, their representatives, and their perks, and essentially became tools of the industry. And, if this seemed somewhat abstract during one of Dr. Webber's lectures, the information became crystal clear when one walked through the door entering into the fantasy world of drug day.

Drug day, the fourth Thursday in the main auditorium, at noon, was set aside for pharmaceutical companies to put on display their pharmaceuticals. Samples of various drugs were handed out to interns and residents. These companies had learned that their marketing efforts were rewarded if physicians were targeted and sold. Today the fact of the matter is that pharmaceutical companies spend more than 21 billion dollars a year on promoting and marketing their products, of which about 88 percent is directed at physicians. With approximately 600,000 physicians in active practice this amounts to more than $30,000 spent on each physician. This works when physicians lose their moral compass, a predictable casualty of the medical educational process.

The drug day door was guarded by very large security personnel. These hospital security personnel, who assiduously checked nametags to be certain that the initials MD were behind the name, guarded the door leading to the interior of the auditorium. That naturally left out medical students and nurses who still had a vested interest in the proceedings. These guys never seemed to be happy. Name badges were scrutinized as if this were a submerged, subterranean military complex requiring the highest security. When we were medical students, with name badges that simply had our names without MD, it felt a little like buying beer with a fake ID. We would gather in a crowd of legitimate physicians, with MD behind their names on the name tags, and try to mix in while being carried by the salivating mass into the inner sanctum of drug day. This usually didn't work because these guys had been doing this job for quite a while, they knew all of the tricks, and it seemed that they enjoyed a certain vicarious pleasure in busting us. So, when the day came that we could have MD behind our name on the name tags, the gift of pomposity was suddenly bestowed upon us, we became somewhat obstreperous, and sallied through the checkpoint with smugness and attitude. Once inside the door, the reality of drug day jumped out and demanded attention. Here was a surreal, carnival-like, conglomeration of pharmaceutical companies, arranged side-by-side, in a square, around the auditorium floor. Each company had its best products on display, with energized representatives breathlessly hawking their wares to physicians-in-training.

So, while we had been warned about the predatory behavior of the sellers of drugs, while we had been warned by Dr. Webber, this was theoretical at the time, we were just dipping our toes into the health care drama; but, within a short period of time the real world would be let loose on us.

While physicians-in-training were making the rounds of the different booths, a gaggle of medical students, student nurses, and nurses hung around the main door. From time to time a rendezvous took place between a harried intern or resident and one of our congregation at the door. Two of the most cherished items were amphetamines, marketed as diet pills, but which actually were used to stay up day and night when on call, and birth control pills, which had revolutionized social behavior. These samples were given away without discretion, simply for the asking, leaving a subtle and indelible imprint in the minds of the young doctors, an imprint which would influence the ordering practices of these future practitioners.

This was what Dr. Webber was so concerned about, what fueled his passion and prescience regarding the fledgling industrial-pharmaceutical complex; an industry, which promised to grow in influence, with an eye towards a self-serving direction of health care, where avarice eclipsed professionalism.

Dr Webber helped us understand how physicians, and their drug ordering practices, have been like ping pong balls, batted around between the pharmaceutical industry and the FDA during the past 100 years. The FDA dates its birth during the presidency of Theodore Roosevelt, and was given its impetus by Dr. Harvey Wiley. During the past 100 years it has been a classic battle between liberal idealists, whose mandate has been to recruit the federal government to allow the FDA powers to protect consumers against dangerous drugs, verses business interests, who have appealed to conservative politicians to allow individuals to make their own choices. As always, politics has become embedded within the fray, obfuscating the issues, substituting ideology for careful thinking. Because careful analysis and thinking is in short demand regarding pharmaceuticals, we young doctors were cannon fodder for the political process. The FDA developed a methodology based on the scientific method, to ferret out dangerous and untested drugs. Today, however, all is not well with the FDA. What has evolved is a tenuous détente between the FDA and pharmaceutical companies, which has some dangerous implications for gullible physicians.

Performance-enhancing drugs, now an issue with major league baseball, sheds some light on this troubling situation. In 1995, shortly after the baseball strike of 1994, legislation sailed through congress, which required the FDA to prove that an herb or supplement was not safe or efficacious, rather than that being a requirement of the herbal manufacturer. In this instance, business prevailed over government and with a snap of the legislative finger, herbs, vitamins, and supplements became available over the counter, without a prescription, and the flood gates were opened for performance enhancing items like androstenedione, a first cousin of anabolic steroids, and now a scourge for major league baseball. So while anabolic steroids were outlawed in 1998, these over-the-counter pills are still legal, a major problem for baseball team owners, baseball players and their union, and the fans whose children often emulate their heroes of the diamond.

Today, much of the scientific literature and many of the authors are in some way connected to the drug companies, which provides financial support to the investigators at the same time opening the way for subtle bias; a stealth influence upon practicing physicians who have traditionally assumed that reputable medical journals are sacrosanct, free of industry influence, a safe haven. This subtle bias has crept into the fabric of medical meetings where, shortly after presenting the speaker's credentials, there is a now the disclosure information, which in a perfunctory and brief manner submits to the audience the financial relationship between the authors and drug companies. This information is in fine print, a brief disclaimer that rarely reaches the radar of consciousness.

The FDA can count amongst its reviewers and scientists members who have financial ties to drug companies. All of this creates a dangerous landscape for physicians learning about new pharmaceuticals, but who are vulnerable to the sophisticated marketing techniques that take less effort than carefully reviewing the science, a sad state of affairs. Dr. Webber couldn't have known about this development, but he was savvy enough to wonder, to warn us about the growing influence of the pharmaceutical industry.

I must confess that I have been an easy mark for these sophisticated marketing techniques. I am still encouraged to adhere to a particular prescribing pattern that favors this or that drug company. It is all so seductive. It is so much easier to learn the proper dose and indication for a drug from an attractive rep than from the literature. Drug day was the beginning of the process of distancing myself from the ethics of healing. It is one of the ways we physicians have lost our way. We have succumbed to an easier, softer way, selling out our power of the pen.. The pharmaceutical industry has become emboldened and continues to apply the heat by redirecting promotional and advertising efforts directly to the public thanks to congressional legislation passed in 1995. Now, patients demand the glitzy drugs they learn about while watching television. The pressure is great, but physicians and legislators have opened the floodgates, and we patients have stood silently by. Drug day was simply a commercial effort for predatory marketing, putting these glitzy drugs and future prescribing agents, the doctors, together in a large auditorium, all of which was sanctioned by the training program.

Let's return to the bus illustration I used in the first chapter. You will recall my consternation with the public bus, which advertised a total body CT scan as a legitimate way to ensure good health, much as the patent medicine salespersons did in the 19th century. I have witnessed how the FDA's rather cavalier attitude towards insuring that medical devices have been adequately tested for safety and efficacy contributes mightily to this consternation. Medical devices are released for clinical use long before meaningful data has been generated attesting to their usefulness. It is one thing to use a drug off label, i.e. in a way not yet approved by the FDA, yet where there is some scientific evidence which supports this behavior, but quite another to use a device on a patient that has not been thoroughly and rigorously tested. This is not unusual. Many of the devices now part of our arsenal are incompletely tested, not fully and rigorously assessed in long term random clinical trials. As a gastroenterologist I have seen how that has played out with endoscopic devices. The gastric balloon, which was purported to facilitate weight loss in patients with morbid obesity, is a good example. Although not essential to life, the stomach nevertheless is a very important organ. The stomach acts like a reservoir, a receptacle that churns and prepares food for delivery into the small intestine where the job of digestion occurs. There are enzymes, which in its acid milieu allows the stomach to make food into a paste in preparation for digestion. The acid environment helps prevent infectious organisms gaining access to the digestive tract and wrecking havoc. Yet, the stomach is a relic of the past. Before there were McDonald's Golden Arches on every corner, the stomach allowed Homo sapiens to store food and make it ready for use during those lengthy periods between meals, which were part of our early nomadic existence. So, with little respect for the stomach's contribution to the success of our species, with disdain and irreverence, the FDA approved the use of the gastric balloon, which was to fill the stomach with an inert object, feigning satiety, limiting the space for the early preparatory steps of digestion, and leading to weight loss. Unfortunately, it was released too soon, before it was adequately tested and predictably there were significant complications. Another example is the total hip replacement. The hip joint is composed of the acetabulum, a cup-like extension emanating from the pelvis and the ball-like configuration of the femur, which nicely fits into the acetabulum. This gives us the ability to benefit from bipedal locomotion, a evolutional development that we take for granted; but not if osteoarthritis invades the joint. The precise fitting of the femur into the acetabulum is distorted by irregularities caused by osteoarthritis on the surfaces of the joint, causing pain and suffering. Orthopedic surgeons have become expert in total hip replacements, where their surgical expertise has led to developing and surgically installing a metal ball into a plastic cup. In 2005 a modification was introduced, which led to a new metal-on-metal design in which both components were made from a metal alloy. The devise was hastily approved by the FDA. It was soon apparent that this new devise failed at the rate of at least one in eight. This was a tragedy for many patients and the devise was recalled. Mind you, the FDA's laxity in this area simply plays into the hands of technophysicians who are surveying the horizon for lucrative procedures.

But the dreaded spotlight falls on those over eager technophysicians who rush to be the first on the block, running through red lights, oblivious to potential complications, with the usual perfidious motivations. And, there were any number of complications with these devices, complications that laid bare the insolence of the device manufacturers, but more importantly, physicians, like myself, whose focus was mostly self serving.

James T. Hansen, M.D.

Clinical trials are where new drugs and devices are tested on live patients, after the basic research attests to their general safety, and after preliminary trials with surrogate animals, and ultimately patients, have validated the hypothesized efficacy and safety. These studies have traditionally been carried out in medical schools with faculty supervision and participation. I know that Dr. Webber would be dismayed by the evolution of the clinical trial. More recently, as the number of clinical trials has increased, in part because of the increased number of new drugs and devices, pharmaceutical companies have found that technophysicians are ready and willing partners, anxious to participate in these trials because the pay is good. It is easier for private technophysicians to recruit the requisite number of participants because they are more intimate with the patients, and patients prefer more comfortable surroundings than in a large tertiary hospital. So, patients are enrolled in these studies, usually paid, and permission is obtained from the hospital's Institution Review Committee, which is charged with insuring that the study is ethical and safe. The IRC is usually generous and complicit.

In gastroenterology it is an attractive proposition since the role of the gastroenterologist is to perform procedures on patients as part of a clinical trial. A primary investigator with the pharmaceutical company evaluates the data and interprets it. The clinical gastroenterologist simply performs the procedure for a healthy stipend, and does nothing else. Quality control is an issue here. The mercenary gastroenterologist sees this as a financial opportunity, and not necessarily an opportunity to contribute to the research effort. This contributes to sloppy data and questionable results. We have witnessed the number of private-practice physicians engaged in drug studies nearly tripling from about 4,000 in 1990 to more than 11,000 in 1997. Between 1991 and 1998, the percentage of industry money for clinical trials at academic medical centers declined from 80% to 40%. It is quite clear what is happening.

Why do physicians spend their valuable time doing this clinical trial stuff?

As we have already said, between 1995 and 1999 physicians income, adjusted for inflation, fell more than 6%, with the average specialist's income falling by 4%. This was during a time period when salaries and wages rose for most workers. So, it's not rocket science. Money is a major motivator. While health care expenditures have been going up, physicians' incomes have fallen. We technophysicians, who have been loosened from the shackles of meaningful health care, find new ways to supplement our incomes, contributing to the ever rising health care expenditures, while allowing quality to free fall into oblivion. Physicians are entitled to meaningful remuneration, but the ethical boundaries of financial gain are blurred.

While much of the technological advance that has clinical relevance today is initially developed as a result of medical research, much of what we do in the practice of medicine has simply been handed down from one generation of physicians to another, often without a scientific basis. The use of the nasogastric tube comes to mind. This is a tube inserted into the stomach, ostensibly designed to decompress the stomach, remove unwanted secretions, and provide a venue for administering medications. It has been a mainstay in the management of the postoperative patient, felt to prevent vomiting and to hasten healing. Recent studies have brought into question the validity of its use. Pancreatitis is an example where the data reveals that most patients do better without the tube. Science has taken a backward glance and appropriately advised against this treatment. What we have done and often what we do today is often because it has always been done that way. Frankly a great deal of what we do is at best quasi-scientific. During the past century the scientific method has given us more and more tools for the practice of medicine. Today, many new drugs, new tests, new surgical procedures, and new technology are born of scientific investigation. This is especially true today where there is a huge financial stake. With so much faith in science, the scientific method has become a cash cow for investigators, pharmaceutical companies, medical device manufacturers, and those physicians who become expert at using the product. Research physicians become a little like airline pilots with a vast array of switches, monitors, levers, and very minimal contact with the passengers or patients. Part of my training involved learning how to carry out bench research. The supposition is that information eventually flows from the bench to the bedside and that we would be better doctors for knowing this. I was sinking faster and further into the quicksand of science, of the probing, intrusive side of health care. Health care research is often carried out with mammalian surrogates for Homo sapiens. In our program it was to be rats. These helpless rodents have offered up a number of discoveries, which have translated into useful clinical tools.

I hated the damn things. But, why should I hate rats? They have certainly served science well, becoming the substrate for medical experimentation and scientific discovery. When I was in medical school I spent summer time working with these creatures. At that time the task was to find a new diabetic drug, an oral hypoglycemic agent to hopefully replace insulin. My job was to take these large white rats, Sprague Dawley rats, inject them with an agent called alloxane, which destroyed their insulin secreting cells rendering them diabetic, and to treat the animals with a new drug called phenthylbiguanide. I had to grab these squealing, biting, frightened animals by the tail, careful to wear a large glove to protect my hand, and draw blood from the outer canthus of their eyes, or from their tails, to test for glucose. They fought ferociously, they were able to bite through the large glove in spite of its padding, they created so much fury inside of me that on more than one occasion I tossed the goddamn things against the wall ending their misery. I don't think anyone every saw me do it. Not many of them ended up that way and no one kept count of how many rats we had. I was often left alone in one of the rat rooms filled with smog and heat and unhappy rodents.

Still, why should I hate rats. Sure, they were part of the drama of the terrible plague, and they certainly carry disease. Cats gloat when they have killed them, bringing their mangled carcasses to the front door, for all to see their ugliness. Yet, as I look back upon this experience, there is something else. I recalled the battle between the fisherman, Santiago, and the giant marlin in Hemingway's novel, *The Old Man And the Sea*. The old man both loved and loathed the fish with whom he was engaged in mortal combat. The fish's heroic effort, what he gave in this fight for his life, earned respect from the old man. The fish had no choice, given his circumstance, but he performed on this stage with brilliance, struggling to the end, never surrendering. Other than circumstance, there was nothing else the fish could do, but do it well he did. The old man had choice; he could have given up, but he chose not to do so. Even so, why did I hate the rats? I believe it was because, like the fish, the rats had no choice, yet they played out their part with valor, never giving up. They stayed the course. I, on the other hand, blessed with free choice, often took a path, which was self-serving, pragmatic, often without much honor or courage. My path, my journey to become a doctor, invited and encouraged me to be a part of herd mentality, not necessarily honorable or courageous, often doing it like we were told, without protestation. I envied the rats for their commitment, their instinctual struggle to stay alive, without equivocation, their steadfast behavior, their resolve. My free will made it much more difficult to find honor and fulfillment, although I honestly don't believe that those elements had anything to do with the rats or the fish. At the time, these feelings were subliminal, but a lighthouse, beckoning me to a safe harbor.

Much of this research was funded by pharmaceutical companies. Fundamentally, I have come to understand that using surrogate creatures has been extremely important to the advancement of medicine. In one sense, these are animals, they live by automatic pilot, without a soul, albeit the ability to survive by instinct, a learned response. So, in a very subtle way an obligatory covenant was struck between drug companies and those of us working on various projects, as well as physicians in general. Drug companies and biomedical device companies are totally involved in developing their product, which, although leaving mankind somewhat better off, leaves a subliminal contract between the health care profession and themselves. This has led to much mischief.

Even the coffee cups and pens so eagerly dispensed by pharmaceutical reps create a sense of indebtedness. I vividly remember one of the gifts I received from Eli Lilly, a pharmaceutical company. When I graduated from medical school in 1961, like my colleagues I received a black doctor's bag. Although it sounds a little hokey, I was so proud of that thing. I proudly carried it on my first day as an intern, now with MD behind my name, emblazoned on my bag, in spite of the fact that I didn't know very much. My handwriting has always been atrocious, a defining characteristic of many physicians, and so I quickly learned to type my reports when I was on duty. The on call schedule is grueling. Thirty six hours on, admitting new patients, relieving their suffering, administering medications, calling in specialists, and trying to maintain an even keel. I remember the patient. He was in the admitting area, lying quietly in a metal framed bed, a face pinched because he was edentulous, without teeth, eye lids at half mast, disheveled, incoherent, and fairly typical of many of our patients at Los Angeles County General Hospital. I carefully examined him, using the shiny instruments in my new black doctor's bag. After I finished I proceeded to the intern-resident room to type my report. I was so full of myself. I left my black bag beside the patient to remind him of my station, that help was present, that I was a trained professional. When I finished typing I walked back into the admitting room to move to the next patient who needed my help. I anxiously looked forward to gathering up my badge of honor, my black bag, and evaluating this next patient. What I saw stopped me in my tracks. Clearly an invisible hand was subtly adjusting my grandiosity. When I reached for my new black doctor's bag,

James T. Hansen, M.D.

I saw a glimpse of Hades. There, sharing space with my new stethoscope, reflex hammer, and ophthalmoscope, was a sea of urine, spittle, and feces. My patient had used my new black bag as his personal toilet. My new instruments were floating in this rude medium, an assault on modern medicine, this cesspool.

I stood still for a few moments, not sure what to do, glancing at the patient who was snoozing and oblivious of the moment's catastrophe. I did the only thing that made sense to me. I gingerly grasped the handles of my new black doctor bag, walked over to the nearest receptacle, dropped my bag in and said farewell. I have never had another doctor bag. In retrospect, I believe this was the ghost of an ultimate healer who was admonishing me for accepting a gift from a pharmaceutical company, a gift designed to buy my future prescriptions.

The picture that emerges here is a profession that readily accepts gifts, dinners, and free continuing education. Even though the extent of physician involvement with industry is not made public, evidence suggests that a great many are collaborating, and that many have financial deals with multiple companies. It reveals a profession heavily involved with helping industry market its products with speaking engagements, ghostwritten articles, and in regulatory deliberations. It illustrates how some physicians exploit their professional standing to promote their own financial well being over the best interest of their patients. All of this serves to harm patients and increase the cost of care. Without moral ballast, without an ethical rudder, physicians are cannon fodder for the marketing and promotional efforts of the pharmaceutical industry. It is so easy to assuage one's self that this is science, that it is acceptable behavior for those of us who are privileged to write prescriptions, to order tests, to do procedures or surgeries, because we are medical doctors and are blessed by the gods on Mount Olympus. This is unacceptable behavior. The ghost of Dr. Webber cries out. `

So it is with the unhealthy alliance between physicians and the pharmaceutical industry. It is a piece of the larger picture, of physicians adrift in a sea without a moral compass, grabbing on to the driftwood of illusion and false promises, without accountability for those of us who need help from a professional we can trust.

The center of my universe now shifted from Los Angeles to Sacramento. This was to be the place where I would spend nearly 30 years, the major period of my career, and where wisdom eventually grew by accretion. Early on I experienced an epiphany of sorts, a sentinel event that ultimately led to an inexorable change in my focus and a clearer perception of reality. The story of Hank had profound implications for me, but it took a while for meaningful assimilation. The lessons I learned in Los Angeles were scrutinized, dissected, and reformulated, leaving a faint trail of uncertainty.

Chapter 6
The Angels Mourn: An Avoidable Loss

The central valley of California is a fantastically fertile stretch from the Tehachapi Mountains to Lake Shasta. It is a veritable garden where much of the world's produce is grown. The summer heat is oppressive, trapped as such in an inversion layer, and a reminder of nature's unadulterated harshness. In August there are very few reasons why a sane person would be standing outside. But there I was. And, I wasn't alone.

A deathly silence was broken by the first of an avalanche of half-empty beer cans hurled into the grave. The first one landed with a metallic thud on the closed coffin. Suddenly the air was filled with Budweiser, Coors and Miller, with frothy, golden brew spilling onto the closed lid of the coffin, the cans randomly careening off into the earth of the freshly dug grave. The odor of beer combined with the fresh earth offered a startling jolt to the sense of smell. There was urgency, rebellion, sadness, and the texture of nihilism.

We were standing in a semicircle around the grave, several large, burly men, most of whom had long, scraggly hair, shaggy beards, and faces weathered by the sun, and myself. There were a few women, without makeup, dressed in leathers, whispering amongst themselves. The guys were shuffling their feet, swearing under their breath, spitting, grunting, staring at the ground. The shiny, chrome-appointed motorcycles stood a silent vigil behind us. I had managed to find an inconspicuous place to park my BMW. By now the preacher and the hearse were silently stealing away. This was a biker funeral. Most of these men were Hell's Angels, marked by their characteristic leather vests and provocative tattoos. These people were saying good by to a buddy, a guy named Hank, a guy I had come to know well.

The Hell's Angels have changed considerably since they were born shortly after World War II in Fontana, California. Initially a group of restless fighter pilots with nothing but time on their hands, filled with wanderlust and a passion for speed, they have become outlaws heavily involved in the manufacture and distribution of another type of speed-- methamphetamine. A peculiar blend of nationalism and anti - government sentiment forms an adhesive bond amongst the members. Territorial, protective of their women, lifestyle, and space, the Angels possess sophisticated weaponry and the will to enforce. Hank was a Hell's Angel.

I met Hank in November 1973. He was 31 years old, a laborer, married with an eleven-year-old daughter. Hank was one of the first patients that I saw in private practice. He had been hospitalized for a couple of days in November with a recurrence of his peptic ulcer disease. This seemed fairly straight forward. I was asked to see him in consultation. I was now the new gastroenterologist in a multispecialty group of internists and I was flushed with pride, power and stature. I had spent a long time preparing for this moment and I felt very deserving. Now it was for real. Hank had had two previous hospitalizations at Memorial Hospital for his ulcer disease, which he didn't help by a lifestyle of smoking and drinking. These had occurred before I had come to town.

Memorial Hospital was a small propriety hospital built and owned by a group of physicians. It was in the north part of town, a rough area, and its reputation was a point of discussion. It was a small for- profit hospital with a marginal group of general practitioners who accounted for most of the admissions many of whom were on welfare. This was the least progressive of the hospitals in town, a barebones operation, with just the basics, yet, profitable ! The medical staff was anxious to attract bright new specialists and provide them with whatever equipment or technology they wanted. I had been welcomed with open arms.

The surrounding neighborhood was predominantly black, medically underserved, and burdened by crime and drugs. The nursing staff was primarily black and Hispanic. There had been employee grievances against the all white physician ownership but I was unaware of the details. There were apparently some civil rights issues, which had gotten the attention the NAACP. At that point none of this affected my life in the least. I was the new gastroenterologist. I remember walking down the hallway to meet Hank. I was the center of my universe with a brand new sport coat, white shirt, tie, and freshly polished shoes. The feelings were not so dissimilar from the first day I put on my long white coat. The nurses still wore caps then and seemed appropriately deferential. I smiled back filled with supreme confidence. I was already busy seeing patients in several other hospitals, churning out those procedures that separated me from the rest and promised the good life. God, I was hot shit!

It broke through my manufactured calm like a howitzer. Out of nowhere came that little piece of paper that fundamentally changed my life. It came in the mail, not totally unexpected, but an insult to my well honed take of myself. It took my artfully crafted homeostasis and stood all of that manufactured tranquility on its head. This summons and complaint was a fundamental assault on my take of self worth. Someone, an attorney, had the audacity to suggest that I had mishandled a case, that my best was wanting, guilty of substandard practice, responsible for a failing grade. That had never happened to me. My heart soared into my throat, my senses jumbled, my consciousness assaulted--there was nothing else I could concentrate on. Angry and frightened at the same time, I wasn't sure who to strike out against, only that there must some potential target. I wasn't even on call that fateful night. Why had the telephone exchange called me?

I found the doctor's dinning room to be a safe refuge. Every hospital has a doctor's dining room. Slowly becoming anachronistic, they were the center of the health care universe when physicians had more power and control. It was a watering hole where physicians gathered to reinforce the status quo. The most luxurious, most tastefully appointed room in the hospital, where physicians gathered to enjoy the hospital's best food and to unwind. A place where referrals were made, physician leadership positions selected, the performance of the hospital administrator discussed, where physicians were free to unleash vitriol directed towards the government, patients, and attorneys. Malpractice attorneys have been the bane of physicians as long as I have been in the business, and long before that. They are bright, medically savvy, and more than willing to impugn the integrity of any physician caught in the cross hairs of a malpractice action. Like a nightmare. Nearly every physician has had some experience with this species. So, when I shared my woes in the doctor's dining room there were any number of colleagues who had advice and were willing to sympathize.

The news of the malpractice suit, the death of Hank, spread through the hospital with the speed of light. I had just finished lunch when Phil

O'Brien, the chief of staff, sat down beside me and asked "How are you handling things, Jim?" The table was cluttered with dirty dishes, sandwich wrappers, empty soft drink cans, and condiments smeared here and there. Several physicians were busy reading the Wall Street Journal and a couple of surgeons, dressed in their characteristic "greens", were snoring in reclining chairs. The hospital PA system was fully engaged calling for this and that doctor, some of whom roused themselves from their reverie to pick up the phone. The sound of the air conditioning unit provided baleful background music.

Somewhat naively, I responded " I'm not sure what to do?"

O'Brien shot back, "just do what your attorney says. Just keep your head up."

About this time Cliff Winston joined us. He was portly and obnoxious. He had plethoric features with a large bulbous nose, a thin mustache, and frontal balding. He seemed to be enveloped by a peculiar, offensive odor wherever he went. Cliff was the hospital's pathologist and he knew all about the unplanned end of Hank's life. He had had a number of malpractice experiences himself and it was said that he was lucky not to be in the slammer. "Hansen, they'll try to fuck you over. They know that you're green and they can smell the big bucks. Shakespeare was right--all these goddamn lawyers should be hung."

O'Brien continued, "Jim, you did what you could. This type of patient doesn't take care of himself. These guys never work, they're on welfare, they're non compliant, and they just suck the system dry. If the guy hadn't been a drinker and smoker chances are that he would have never been in the hospital in the first place." As several physicians walked to the cafeteria tray line they patted me on the shoulder, shaking their heads, and whispering to each other. I felt terrible. There had been worse fuck-ups in training but somehow the university always covered my ass. My attorney asked me to write out a complete narrative of the case, not to put it into the patient's chart, not to talk with any of the family, and gird myself for interrogatories where difficult questions would be asked by the opposing side. My take of him was that he was too anxious to agree with our side of the story, at least the side of the story that the hospital endorsed, too ready to believe anything I said. All of this left me a little unnerved. The medical staff didn't take any action against me so I could continue to practice. The bylaws contained a ton of verbiage to protect the doctor until he was judged incompetent, impaired, or guilty of a felony. It occurred to me that this might allow bad doctors to continue to put patients at risk while the matter moved through the labyrinthine process of peer review. Christ, was I a bad doctor?

Hank was actually a fairly pleasant guy. He did have a job. He had been a carpenter but was now a general laborer. His wife was named Pam. He liked to fish and hunt and, of course, ride his bike. He had been married twice before. I suppose that you would have called his wife a "mama". Hank taught me that a biker "mama" is fiercely monogamous, very protective of her man, not adverse to resorting to physical means to protect what was hers. By contradistinction, a "critter" was a new female in the group. "Critters" tended to be polygamous, forever a source of ire to the "mamas", and destined at some point to become a "mama". I didn't know if all of this was actually true but it was interesting conversation. Hank' father had died of a heart attack and he had a brother who was killed in Viet Nam.

Hank had an upper GI series during that short November admission which revealed an ulcer. He responded to conservative therapy and was discharged after seven uneventful days. This would have probably been a one or two day hospitalization today, or even an outpatient event, but in 1974, when even MediCal was paying on a fee-for-service basis without many questions, a one week's stay in an expensive hospital bed for a stable patient was the norm. We all bitched about the government's discount of our fee, but we just saw more patients and didn't pay too much attention to the length of stay. Very lucrative!

I first met Stuart Jackson at the dreaded interrogatory. I didn't know much about him but simply seeing and hearing him demanded that I know more about this guy. Stuart Jackson had become a charter member of black attorneys who had cut their teeth during the civil rights movement in the 1960s. The lunch counter in Carolina, the bus strike in Montgomery, and the march in Selma gave birth to a number of articulate, brave, driven black men who took the law, the Constitution, and the Bill of Rights seriously.

The 1954 Brown v. The Board of Education decision unleashed a fury of passion tempered by the legacy of Ghandi and Dr. King's admonition for civil disobedience. Stuart Jackson was the real thing, authentic, honed during the tumultuous civil rights struggle, and a hell of an adversary. Some of this I learned during the interrogatory.

Mr. Jackson was always courteous, charming, and this was disarming. I later learned from an attorney friend that he took the case because he had it out for Memorial Hospital. He was convinced that there were some unfair hiring practices, that minorities were being held to a different performance standard, a different pay schedule, and different types of discipline. Since the hospital was a co-defendant I found myself in his line of fire. There were several other physicians involved, but none intimately involved with order writing, now a testament to the technophysician in me. Naturally I had gone over all of my records with a fine tuned comb and everything I thought important, everything my attorney thought important, was committed to memory. I had seen Hank on several occasions before that last admission of July 3, 1974. Thank God for progress notes, thank God I had learned to write everything down, thank God I had learned that lesson well. I was so busy, so many patients to see, so many consultations, so many hospitals to make rounds in, so many elective procedures, so many call nights to see patients in the ER or ICU. The money was great and the main reason I put up with all this shit. This was inhuman but greed had taken over. I think that I worked harder that first year in private practice than I ever did in training.

The interrogatory took place in my office. My world. I have learned that this is not so unusual. Although I was the defendant, I think the trick was to put me at ease, let me savor the trappings of power, sort of lull me into complacency. It didn't actually work in my case since Mr. Jackson was so imposing, since I was so frightened, since my self worth was now melting. I had worked so hard to build a facade of approval. The only way I could glean who I actually was was to mirror my persona in the faces and behavior of the world that I touched. If someone came at me sideways, if I sensed disapproval, I was devastated.

We were all ready. My attorney, fashioned to a T with his pin striped suit of armor, classically waspish; the court reporter, a smallish woman in her fifties, wearing a pleated skirt with a frilly pastel blouse, a gravelly voice, very proper. And, Mr. Jackson, standing nearly 6'3", robust, attired in a three piece charcoal grey summer suit, a large cigar in his front pocket, and a gold watch dangling from vest pocket. The hospital attorney was also present. Decked out in a tan polyester summer suit, he was basically non nondescript, furiously taking notes and saying very little. The door was closed, the office staff was instructed to hold all incoming calls and to leave us alone. That was scary. Cut off from the world, sitting on the proverbial hot seat, left to marinate in my own juices--not a pleasant feeling.

My attorney, Scott Hightower, made the formal introductions in a curt, officious voice. He was obviously nervous and the bonhomie that developed between us faded. Mr. Jackson walked over to my desk, towered above me, and shook my hand. There are times in one's life when the sheer power of one individual is transmitted by way of a handshake. When I was a medical student, "moonlighting" in Los Angeles, I had the same feeling when I cared for Marion Morrison-I felt eclipsed by his power much as I did with Stuart Jackson. It was an out-of-body experience. But Marion Morrison. Who was he?

As an extern at Good Samaritan Hospital in Los Angeles I earned my room and board by doing the history and physical exams for staff doctors, obviating their need to come to the hospital in the evening with non-critical cases. I was a third year medical student. I am not sure the laws today would allow such an arrangement, but the year was 1964. On that particular night I strode across the street from my quarters to the hospital and picked up my list of patients to see. It was an ordinary night with the usual preoperative patients for gall bladder surgery, colon resections, and the last on my list, Marion Morrison for a lung resection. As I approached the nursing station, there was some apprehension on the faces of the nurses on duty. I asked for and was given the chart. It seemed to me that their apprehension related to my seeing a cancer patient, something I had already done, and not a problem. No words were spoken, but these nurses seemed so up tight. I strode down the hall to Morrison's room, knocked and entered. It hit me between the eyes; this was unexpected. There in this hospital bed was someone bigger than life, but at the moment I could not recall his name. His first words were "come on in, Doc." The voice was unmistakable, now I knew who it was; this was John Wayne. I was petrified. I introduced myself, with a cracking voice, my knees weak, uncertainty and timidity betraying the moment. He called his wife in from an adjoining room with that unmistakable voice. I tried to wrap the blood pressure cuff around his huge arm, my hands were shaking; but he helped me, saving my ass and reducing my stress at least a modicum. No sooner than I entered, I was gone. My moment with this giant was a fleeting one, buried in my memory bank, but momentarily dusted off when I met Mr. Jackson.

Stuart Jackson's hand was also huge, powerful, and warm. For a brief second I was totally engulfed by this great man, much as I had been with John Wayne. His eyes never left mine. The thought occurred to me that this might be a good time to ask for an autograph but common sense returned when I realized that this guy was out to fry my ass. So I remained frozen behind my desk, feeling stupid, insipid at best, not certain what I should do next.

"Pleased to meet you, Dr. Hansen", Mr. Jackson smiled.

I could only mutter "thank you." I wanted to say more but my mouth was dry and parched and the effort of breathing took precedence at that moment. We all settled in our seats. The attorneys and court reporter were in straight backed chairs while I timidly sank in my cushioned swivel chair. Mr. Jackson nodded to the court reporter, who instinctively set up her machine. A little like a typewriter, but smaller, and with different keys, within a short period of time it became an adversary. When I ultimately read the transcript several weeks later I realized that every word was recorded, even the "uhs, ohs", and most other unflattering verbal sounds.

There were some perfunctory introductions. The court reporter began to work. Mr. Jackson then turned his attention to me and, for the record, asked me to spell my full name, place or birth, educational background, and professional qualifications. He then surprised me by musing that I sounded more like an expert witness than a defendant. I'm not sure what that meant. I accepted it as flattery but I wondered. Mr. Jackson's voice filled the room with a deep and sonorous fragrance. We all sat transfixed when he talked. Each phrase was a soliloquy. He spoke from deep within himself, betraying the depth of his experience, inviting us to feel the wounds of his words born from the civil rights battlefield.

I was asked to recount my involvement with Hank. Although well prepared, my voice cracked. I found it difficult to put a complete sentence together. I recalled my first meeting with Hank in November, 1973, while he was hospitalized. I saw Hank three subsequent times in the office. As an outpatient he had been doing well on medication but in May his abdominal pain returned. He was hospitalized in June by his family physician and shortly thereafter operated upon by a general surgeon, all of whom were in the cross hairs of this malpractice suit. I was a little pissed that I wasn't asked to see him before that decision was made. In July, while he was a postoperative patient, I was asked to see him for the last time. He suffered from intractable nausea and vomiting.

I could hear myself speaking. Like that proverbial nightmare where some person is coming after you everything moved in slow motion and I couldn't get away. I could hear breathing and a few scattered coughs, mostly from the court reporter, but nothing else except my voice and my heart pounding. From time to time I referred to my notes but I didn't actually need them. Mr. Jackson sat still with a benevolent countenance, never betraying what he was thinking, his eyes guiding me in a professorial manner. I continued.

I learned that Hank had an obstruction in the area of the surgical anastomosis, the connection between the edges of the resection, where these edges were sutured together, maintaining continuity. This was apparent from barium x-rays. I went ahead and scoped Hank to discern whether this was a mechanical obstruction or a functional one, perhaps caused by a lazy postoperative stomach. The procedure revealed edema at the site of the surgical anastomosis, a functional blockage of the flow of ingested food. My treatment plan included continuous nasogastric suction, with that tube that is now nearly obsolete, to decompress his stomach and intravenous fluids. He was very slow to improve and it was clear that he needed nutritional support. One of the tools in my box was the ability to insert a subclavian catheter and to administer hyperalimentation. The catheter was passed percutaneously, blindly, and its position in the larger superior vena cava, a large vein that empties into the heart, was verified by x-ray. This is a dangerous procedure with many possible complications if not done properly but I knew what I was doing and I was successful. Hyperalimentation, also called total parental nutrition, was a relatively new technique in 1973. A solution loaded with protein and glucose was administered through this catheter and allowed us to nutritionally sustain Hank without burdening his impaired stomach.

As I recounted the details I was confronted with memories of Hank. He was a good patient, a little weird, totally absorbed by his motorcycle, language born of the road, completely trusting my ministrations. My moments with Hank were brief but we developed a working relationship. Memorial Hospital was out of my beaten path and I usually made rounds there at the end of the day. This was not infrequently during the early evening hours. During that first year of private practice my pager smoked with any number of calls. Since I was the only gastroenterologist in the group it was not uncommon for me to have to go back to one of the other hospitals where I had already been to see an emergency patient, usually a patient with a gastrointestinal bleed. Although bone tired, the rewards were substantial and everyone expected me to do a procedure. There was never much thought given to alternative approaches. Seduced by technology, procedures became second nature even though I learned that the vast majority of these patients stopped bleeding with simple bed rest. Never mind. The hospital industry, the endoscope manufacturers, the referring physicians, and the patients expected the best. Much as Evans revealed to me, it had become a birthright. And I bought the whole ball of wax. On the other hand, the alternative, not to have done what I did, would have also been scrutinized with an eye towards litigation, as this was an avoidable death.

Hank was easy to talk to. I am sure that conversation was a luxury for him. He spent his days on his back with the omnipresent nasogastric tube and the subclavian catheter, a conduit of life sustaining fluid. He was totally out of control, he had relinquished that control because he implicitly trusted me, and I'm not certain how often he had visitors. My impression was that his only visitor was his wife and that these were fairly short visits. Our conversations were usually perfunctory. "How are you feeling, Hank? Do you have any pain? Are you passing any gas? Are you getting out of bed?" I would briefly examine him after glancing at the chart.

What interested me most were his vital signs, his weight, his fluid intake and output, and his blood chemistries. I spent less than 30 seconds digesting this information. I was so tired and usually in a rush. I rarely asked the nurses how he was doing. The evening nurses were usually from some weird third-world country and I couldn't understand them anyway. Hank would invariably ask "Doc, when do I get out of this fucking place? Doc, you ought to check out the head nurse during the day. She's got the biggest tits I've ever seen. You think you could order her to spend more time with me?" It occurred to me that I ought to make rounds during the day.

Mr. Jackson listened patiently. My attorney had very little to do. Jackson was particularly interested in how this happened under my nose. Jackson asked, " Dr. Hansen, what did you make of the falling serum sodium ?" I had given that much thought. The guys in the doctors dining room asked me the same thing. That problem had been on my mind those final two weeks. I often had lunch with John Wallace. Wallace was an internist, about mid forties, always impeccably dressed, possessed by the notion that surgeons made too much money, that he actually worked much harder, that it wasn't fair. Wallace had managed to corner the market on reading all of the EKGs in the hospital. That job would ordinarily go to a cardiologist but there were none on the staff and it was said that Wallace had run a couple off to protect his enterprise On more that one occasion I munched a sandwich with him and shared my consternation about Hank' sodium. At the time he seemed like the only person who might understand. Wallace's response was to give him more sodium, but I really didn't trust his judgment. I felt that I was handling that part, and I was mostly interested in the pathophysiologic mechanism that underlay the hyponatremia. I did not give him added sodium.

Wallace would say, "Jim, what's the big deal! He's young, he has good kidneys, he'll ultimately correct himself." In some ways I admired his pragmatism. He wasn't encumbered with the need to know all of the underlying mechanisms. He seemed willing to relinquish some of his control. I had real difficulty with that. Control was an issue for me. I not only needed to manage every aspect of the case but I had a written order to cover every aspect of Hank' existence. I left nothing to chance, almost nothing, as I reflect back upon the serum sodium. I could accept nothing as "the way things were", I micromanaged every aspect of Hank' life and wrested control from him. But that serum sodium?

Stuart Jackson led me towards Hank's final days. I misjudged Jackson and asked him "is all of this detail necessary?" Jackson sat still, engulfing me in his not inconsiderable gaze, glanced at my attorney who seemed mortified, and responded "Dr. Hansen, a young man seems to have died under your care and I believe that you are singularly responsible." That shot through me like a knife. I halfway expected my attorney to object but he didn't. Instead, we took a break and he politely informed me to answer all of Mr. Jackson's questions truthfully. Whose side was this fuck on?

I was nearly at my wit's end. I hadn't slept well since the Summons. I eased my pain with my friend, Jack Daniels. This Hank thing assumed a mosaic pattern in my mind, my thought processes, my dreams. It invaded every aspect of my life. I had trouble concentrating on matters at hand. I was convinced that even if I were found not guilty in this matter Jackson had caught me in a web that would eventually lead me into some other medical disaster. But deep inside, I knew that I was ultimately responsible, that something terrible had gone wrong, that my efforts were subpar. Feelings of responsibility are part of being a doctor. It is part of the mantle of credibility, authenticity, and mystery that drapes our shoulders when we take the Hippocratic Oath.

Jackson continued to dwell on the sodium issue. "Dr. Hansen, what did you do about the falling serum sodium?" I took him through the exhaustive number of tests I ordered in an effort to figure it out. Most of this evaluation was boilerplate—how to evaluate hyponatremia. I had had very little time to clearly think things through and at least the tests would leave the impression that I was in control. There were any number of blood tests, urine tests, x-rays, and nuclear scans. I knew that the nasogastric suction was robbing him of some sodium but I was confident that this was being replaced by the hyperalimentation.

I recalled for Mr. Jackson Hank' final several days. I had gone over all of this with my attorney but under Stuart Jackson's interrogation a spell was cast and more facts emerged. My attorney looked puzzled by these revelations but he also seemed mesmerized by Stuart Jackson. I continued, "Hank seemed a little more withdrawn towards the end. He seemed distant." I remembered calls from the day nurses who were worried that he was depressed. I even had a psychiatrist see him and his impression was that Hank was suffering from a depressive neurosis. Valium was ordered. He became more restless, anxious, but alert and oriented. On the day before he died Hank' kidney function began to fail; his blood urea nitrogen went up. Why were his kidneys failing? This was puzzling. He was putting out urine. He was not on nephrotoxic medicines. He was afebrile. His urinanalysis was normal. The BUN wasn't terribly high but it was still a worry. But I knew what happened and I needed to come clean. I led Mr. Jackson through that last night, a terribly frightening journey, and a terribly frightening task.

On the evening of July 26, a Friday, I made rounds as usual. The drive to Memorial Hospital was tedious because I had to contend with the evening traffic. I had several patients to see and I saved Hank until last. He seemed fine except from time to time there were little involuntary jerking movements. His hyperalimentation was infusing well. His nasogastric tube was functioning well. His physical exam was otherwise normal. The day's lab work had not yet been delivered to the hospital. I told Hank that I was going to be off for the weekend and he replied "don't do anything I wouldn't do, Doc." That gave me a lot of leeway, knowing Hank.

That night I went out for dinner. Several bottles of wine later I was at ease and secure in the knowledge that one of the other guys was covering my practice. I hit the sack around midnight. At 2:00 AM I got a frantic call from the hospital. Since I wasn't on call I wasn't sure why they were calling me but it was about Hank. The nursing staff was concerned that he was intermittently hyperventilating and from time to time seemed unresponsive. Yet, his vital signs were stable and everything else seemed in order. I said thank you and hung up the phone. I was still under the influence of the wine but my mind gradually cleared. I starting running through all the possible problems and suddenly realized that I had never found out Friday's lab. I called the nursing station back and finally got someone who could speak English. It seemed like an eternity before she found the information and read the values back to me. I was petrified. His sodium had fallen further, the BUN had risen considerably and the serum potassium was 8.8 milliequivalents per 100cc of plasma.

That was a lethal value! I had a difficult time computing all of this and then putting a complete sentence together but I eventually gave her some orders to get the potassium down. I hung up the phone and tried to pull myself together. I couldn't wait any longer. I called back. The nurse told me that he was completely unresponsive. She was worried. Instinctively, I got out of bed, still woozy, threw on my clothes, and rushed to the hospital. If he was dead what did I think I would accomplish? What good was it to arrive at this point? I sped on. It is now clear to me that I wanted to look concerned, to look like I was in control, to cover my ass. But, I wasn't in control.

I screeched to a halt in the doctor's parking lot. Usually filled with BMWs, Mercedes, and Porches, it was completely empty. The night air was warm and very still. There were only a couple lights flickering in the hospital. There were no traffic noises only the noise of my breathing. I hurried past the security guard into the hospital and bounded up the stairs to the third floor. No time to wait for the damn elevator. Suddenly I was at the nursing station. There were two women sitting and sobbing--Hank' wife and mother. They barely looked at me but when they did there were looks of scorn. I immediately went with the charge nurse into Hank' room. It was so still. Hank lay quietly in bed. He was dead.

Not knowing what else to do I looked over the equipment that until now had controlled his life. Yet, it didn't really control his life after all, he was gone, things were clearly out of my hands. I still fought that notion and looked for an answer. What had gone wrong? Had I been lulled into deadly compliancy? I turned round and round, desperately wanting to get out of the room, the lights dimmed, only the sounds of sobbing, looking for God knows what. And then, I found it.

Our body fluids have a salinity close to that of sea water which has survived the phylogenetic evolution of our species and stands as a testament to the aquatic origins of Homo sapiens. Our tissues are bathed in a salty solution, sodium chloride, so like the sea, the milieu from which our ancestors crawled many years ago. We are all equipped with bodily mechanisms that maintain the concentration of sodium and chloride within a narrow range that supports life. We carry the sea with us, reminding of us of our legacy, calling to us, never letting us forget our humble beginnings, connecting us to a universal force. It brought to mind the conversation and experience I had with Dan Evans in Mexico.

In 1973 a protein hydrolysate was often used for hyperalimentation. It was enriched with glucose. There were other solutions available, those composed of amino acids, the building blocks of life, and balanced with respect to those important electrolytes, especially sodium and chloride. Not so with the protein hydrolysate. It was one of the first solutions used in hyperalimentation, but primitive. My eyes glanced at the concentration of electrolytes posted on the bottle of protein hydrolysate that had been running into Hank. I remembered his last words to me--don't do anything I wouldn't do. But Hank would not have done this. Right there, in the section that listed the ingredients of the solution, was where I found the answer. The sodium content of the solution was minuscule, certainly not adequate for prolonged hyperalimentation, and begging for additional sodium chloride that one would have normally added to approximate sea water. Hank' falling serum sodium was because he was both losing sodium through the nasogastric tube and not getting enough in the hyperalimentation fluid. This led to subtle but lethal dehydration. No one had picked that up. No one, most of all, me, had taken the time to search for this possibility, not the other doctors nor the nurses. But I was the guy, the new, young technophysician from Los Angeles. Instead, orders were written to do fancy blood tests and x-rays to look for esoteric causes. Tests that were expensive, profitable, and at the same time a convenient substitute for careful thinking. The answer was there plain to see, but obscured by hasty rounds, a casualty of a procedure-oriented focus, a preoccupation with making money. I simply didn't have the time to think carefully through the problem. I saved Memorial Hospital for the end of my rounds, hurrying through these rounds in case there was a lucrative procedure to be done elsewhere, mostly just interested in simply "showing the flag." The ingredient label was there to be seen. My concern for this patient, which was considerable, was eclipsed by the rush to move on, to succumb to my technophysician instincts, rather to any notion of healing.

My office was deathly silent. Mr. Jackson thanked everyone, abruptly stood, surveyed the scene, and left with the others trailing behind. My attorney remained just long enough to tell me that he would be conferring with the other side about a deal. What kind of fucking deal? What had I done? My brief moment of clarity was replaced by rage, insecurity and fear. I began to search for scapegoats. The hospital hadn't provided me with timely lab reports. I wasn't on call when the exchange called. No one else had helped spot the real cause of the low sodium. I had too much to do. God, it went on and on.

I had another moment of clarity as I was leaving Hank' funeral. The air was heavy with the noise of the Harley's awakening to the call of the

Angels. The roar was deafening. In the aggregate it was provocative and frightening-- a bestial disapproval. The workers began filling in the grave. Hank' family had been hidden by the bikers but, crying softly, they were now in plain view, their pain stirred into the mix.

And then they were gone. There was total quiet. The sun blazed, there was no breeze, the dust from the last Harley settled. I came face to face with my powerlessness. I felt terribly vulnerable. Who could I trust? How much control did I really have? Hank became a lab value, a disease entity, a measure of my expertise, not a whole person. I had accepted the notion that his problem was totally amenable to rational thinking, the marvels of science, the dispassion of technology, the lens of a microscope. He was less a person and more a circuit board, only needing some adjustment, simply needing a cure. It was more than just overlooking the inadequate amount of sodium in protein hydrolysate. He could have handed me the clues. There was no time to touch Hank, to listen to him, or to merge with his suffering. This would be inefficient, not productive, requiring more of me than I had available to give. Horseface was looking over my shoulder. I had come to rely on the tonic of high technology because it buffered me from the feelings of the moment, it relieved me of the pain of paradox, it preserved my perception of control. For a moment his death crashed through my solipsism. For just a moment. And then, nothing. Denial raised its ugly head. The pain of this death was so great that I relegated the memory to my subconscious. But it never went away and ultimately helped me see through the veneer of dishonesty that shrouded my technophysician instincts.

Chapter 7
REASON SLUMBERS: Defining Quality

The Hank thing passed; at least the malpractice aspects. I was let off the hook. The hospital was the object of Mr. Colley's focus and it took the hit. I am not sure why I was let off the hook. The emotional evolution, the pain, the self examination, would not have been different even if I had been a party to the settlement. Had I been a party to the settlement it would not have affected my life much since my malpractice insurance would have covered me and the issue would have faded from sight. But my personal anguish was significant and indelible and at least helped me open my eyes. But, time did not stand still. I moved on to other cases, although in retrospect I was a work in progress. I need to jump forward to examine an important topic, one that must be understood to grasp the focus of this book.

Lance Johnson was a 32-year-old man, a huge guy, and an engineer, who worked hard, and managed stress by eating. Using today's standards, he would qualify as morbidly obese. Morbid obesity has become a national epidemic , but in early 1990 this fact was not appreciated. Lance had a major problem. During the course of the day, when demands were coming from all directions, he had a nearly uncontrollable urge to sleep. He was not infrequently found slumped over his desk, snoring, with pencils, papers, and calculators strewn every which way. Driving to and from work was an added chore. He had to fight somnolence every step of the way.

Lance was a nice guy, bright, a good father, and employed by a successful construction firm. His major adversary was falling asleep during the day, a complication of sleep deprivation. Because of his size, and because of difficulty breathing at night, he had what is called sleep apnea. In a recumbent position, the tissues of his larynx and upper airway, being overly sized because of his morbid obesity, collapsed compromising his upper airway. This caused a fall in his blood oxygen saturation, straining his heart, and promising future cardiac difficulties. So, something had to be done.

One of our medical staff's respected ENT physicians saw Lance in consultation and recognized the condition. As part of a routine evaluation he chose to carry out direct laryngoscopy. A tubular device, called a laryngoscope, was inserted into his upper airway to assess his vocal cords and his larynx as part of an evaluation for sleep apnea. The local anesthetic in use for years for this procedure has been cocaine, the same drug that has become a scourge because of its highly addictive nature. Yet, it is a legitimate pharmaceutical, with a long history of use for ENT procedures.

Everything seemed to be going well. The ENT physician and the nurses seemed to be satisfied that the procedure was going well when Lance suddenly had a seizure, then a cardiac arrest, and in spite of an appropriate cardiopulmonary resuscitative effort, he died while being transferred to the hospital's ICU.

The medical executive committee and I, its new president, were presented with a patient who suffered an untoward complication. This was not the kind of thing a new chief of staff likes to cut his teeth on, but there it was. A routine ENT procedure had resulted in the death of a young man. The patient in question was morbidly obese, but that was his only risk factor. This should not have happened. The MEC convened to find out the details of the case and to take appropriate action. There did not seem to be any deviations from the community standard of practice. However, the issue of choosing cocaine over less toxic anesthetics was raised. None of the rest of us knew much about the pertinent literature regarding this subject, but it seemed like a good idea to call a special meeting of the ENT division and discuss these alternative drugs in an effort to seize an opportunity for improvement.

The chair of ENT, who was not a party to the adverse event, summarily dismissed the idea as a waste of time. His response was that all of his colleagues were well trained, understood the value and risk of cocaine, and he was confident that they were well read and were aware of these alternative local anesthetic agents. He didn't see any need for his colleagues to discuss the issue, to examine the literature, to make changes, which might in the future prevent this type of complication.

The MEC's focus was not to indict cocaine, to tell the ENT doctors how to practice medicine, or to mete out punishment. Rather, it was to invite these doctors to brainstorm, to carefully examine their protocols, to look at other prestigious ENT departments and seek out best practice guidelines, and to improve quality. The MEC was stiffed, there was no meaningful information forthcoming from the ENT department, since not many of my colleagues were passionate about this quality business. It was more than slightly frustrating for me, a new chief of staff, filled with idealistic notions of quality management and improvement. The Hank thing had turned me into something akin to a crusader.

This event stands out in my mind because it represents only the tip of the iceberg. My observations have led me to understand that we physicians often have a cavalier attitude about quality, we are happy with their own quality of practice, we don't want anyone nosing around, and we don't see the need for making changes. This short changes the mandate of self-governance. I have come to believe that this attitude is a major player in the health care crisis. This attitude is a lubricant, paving the way for the obscene intrusion of untested gadgets and procedures, the slippery slope of the high technology. Quality has become a casualty of high technology.

The putative overseer of physician issues and behavior in the hospital setting is the Medical Executive Committee. The buck is supposed to stop here. It is composed of the chairs of the various departments, as well as the medical staff officers, and attended by the hospital administrator. This is where medical staff issues are ironed out and where relations with the hospital are kept on track. This is where quality ought to be the central theme—but it's not! Being the medical staff president or chief of staff is a thankless job. Physician agendas are so disparate as to create a quagmire for anyone interested in harvesting the potential strengths that need to be honed. It is akin to herding cats. As the medical staff president, I was aware of a serious complication that had just occurred and because an ENT meeting was out of the question, a special meeting of the MEC was called.

Unfortunately, quality means different things to different people. To some it is the ability to consistently reproduce a product using time-honored methodology. To others, at least in medicine, it is to achieve results with few, if any, complications. To other physicians it is to master the latest technology and to prescribe the latest drugs. And to some it is having additional academic initials behind one's name. Actually, I have come to believe that quality is something quite different and demands to be understood by all as one of the essential areas where a change in attitude is required. My observations and misgivings with quality were harnessed from experiences like Hank and being the Chief of Staff. One of the perks of this office was traveling and learning from workers in the quality field. I thought I had a handle on quality, but I had much to learn.

I have come to learn that quality has more to do with the sequence of events that occur after the patient has accessed the health care system. It is not just related to those activities that lead to cure, but also to those activities that have to do with health maintenance and health restoration. It has to do with the length of time until function is restored. It has to do with appropriate case selection, understanding and balancing quality of life with sanctity of life, and of providing appropriate palliative care. It has to do with length of stay in the hospital, the appropriate transfer to a sub acute or step-down unit, the number of readmissions for the same clinical problem, the number of return visits to the physician for a given problem, and the amount of medication needed to provide symptomatic control. It is not simply the results of basic science investigations. It is not necessarily the data generated by bench research, which focuses on sub cellular or molecular events. Basic science has been and is very important to the clinical practice of medicine but the two are not the same. Quality's measurement requires substantial physician input. Its measurement requires honesty, collaboration, an open mind, and willingness. It invites physicians to subordinate ego and look to published best practice studies which challenge those time honored techniques and style of practice that help define who we are. None of this usually occurs because we physicians are just too busy, and, in fact, the MEC was not much help in dealing with the ENT death.

Quality cries out to be defined for every type of illness, for every disease, for every health maintenance activity. In a sense it is a moving target, as diagnostic and therapeutic endeavors change. This is difficult work, time consuming, and tedious, but I believe that physicians have a moral and ethical responsibility to manage quality, to nourish it, to accept the positive changes by others committed to the process. Physicians willing to make the changes are motivated by their personal commitment to practicing quality medicine. These are physicians who carefully read medical journals, who attend scientific meetings, and who participate in the teaching of health care students. Physicians must be willing to describe their own experience to provide a framework for continuous improvement.

They are the essential ones able to do it. My experience was that it was not happening and it certainly did not happen in Lance's case.

Quality is an important stop on the road to authenticity, a return to common sense medicine, and a halt to spiraling health care expenditures. When quality is not embraced, self-serving behavior supervenes, one of the underpinnings of the technological orgy that many of us physicians have succumbed to. As the Chief of Staff, the inappropriate use of technology, indiscriminate physician ordering practices, and a focus on self interest were there to see and I believe this behavior has contributed significantly to the present health care crisis. I have come to believe that the way out of this debacle is for physicians to look within themselves, to refocus, to dust off that golden kernel of altruism, that Holy Grail, and to embrace quality. This is not asking for new behavior, only to revisit the elements of that basic commitment, an assumption that may not be valid. The evidence is not persuasive that physicians give a whit. So, I have come to believe that it is up to the general public, the consumer, the patient, to insist that there is a behavior change. Without a concerted public effort, single payer medicine or some version of socialized medicine is a guarantee, which I do not believe will solve the problem of embracing quality medicine. True, it may solve the problem of rising expenditures, but quality will be left at the gate. I don't believe that the government has a clue about what happens at the point of service; worse, it doesn't really care. Its interests are primarily fiscal, as long as there are no major health care catastrophes, universal coverage, and of course, being reelected. The health care industry is so ensconced in preserving the present status quo that nothing much can be expected here, at least when it comes with dealing with quality issues in the local hospital. So, don't look for anyone else to deal with this problem. This is a people problem demanding people power. Recall, people power underwrote the success of Act Up, the gay community's advocacy group which focused on speeding up the release of drugs for AIDs. These committed advocates were able to nudge the FDA out of lethargy and make available life saving drugs that were hung up in the approval process. For better or worse, people involved with the Tea Party are committed to undo the Obama health care plan through the political process. In fact, the Obama plan is a response to various political groups that were fed up with insurance underwriting activities, the price of pharmaceuticals, and the unequal access to the heath care industry. People power is available. Many of the societal advances we have seen in this country are a direct result of people power; civil rights, the union movement, amendments to the Constitution, and the outrage over 9/11. It takes citizens, banding together, using mass media, the internet, and a willingness to go to the streets. Thank goodness for the First Amendment.

During my tenure as chief of staff I was rudely awakened to the fact that quality was low down on the totem pole of medical staff interests. In California, like most states, medical staffs are guided by the CMA (or, whatever other state) model staff bylaws when it comes time to create or modify existing bylaws. The bylaws document is the statutory code of behavior that directs physician behavior in reference to medical staff membership. There are a number of elements that constitute any set of bylaws: requirement for membership, election of officers, relationships with the hospital, definition of committees, physician health issues, definition of credentials, the judicial review process and issues of due process, and quality. Nearly 80% of the content of these model bylaws have to due with procedural issues leaving around 20% for quality.

Quality is both ephemeral and elusive. It is not necessarily what someone told you years ago in training, nor what everyone around you is doing. It is fluid, in constant flux, changing as our science becomes more refined. During the golden years of medicine, when there was money aplenty, it was defined, or rather assumed, without regard to cost. Thus, successfully completing a difficult procedure or operation was quality regardless of how much time and resource were consumed. Keeping a dying man alive was quality even though, apart from the moral and ethical considerations, it was quite expensive. There was so much money around for health care, that no one gave it a second thought. Physicians who went through medical school and post graduate training were taught to order every test possible, to embark upon whatever treatment plan was vogue, and not to worry about the dollars.

Quality was assumed to be folded within the lessons that noted physician-teachers taught, what was published in major journals, and whenever high technology was successful in a new endeavor. If a 90 year old man with congestive heart failure was successfully treated with a new medicine, that was quality. If a demanding and difficult surgical procedure, a novel one, was successful in the sense that the patient lived and was discharged from the hospital, that was quality. If a new test, say a technically sophisticated imaging study, provided slightly more information, that was quality. And, if a new drug, perhaps a modification of an existing one, was a bit more effective, that was quality. Quality was often assumed, not defined. If recommendations came out of prestigious medical schools, or were fostered by noted clinicians, that was quality. Finally, the way we did it when we were trained, the lessons we learned early on, were quality. It wasn't terribly important to scrutinize the issue too much since cost was not an issue.

When health care expenditures began to rise, when the dollars became less available, new definitions were needed. Cost became a factor and a new term, value, was given birth. One definition of value is quality divided by cost. Never mind that quality still lacked a clear definition, the expectation was that a good doctor was charged with being a good steward and expected to conserve resources to provide value. Hospitals and payers (insurance companies) now had a vested interest in controlling costs. Quality was subordinated to cost. This is one of the factors that has led to managed care, where providers (a euphemism for doctors) are given a preset amount of money called capitation, defined various ways, ostensibly to control costs, but often to enrich the payers. This then puts the providers at risk, a situation where doctors must practice within the constraints of the prepayment formula, or when the money runs out, take the hit. Cost then became an issue for physicians almost over night. How to define quality continued to be an issue, but now had a price tag. In my opinion, physician reputations are more often based on affability and availability than ability or quality.

As a Chief of Staff, I learned about a number of attempts to define quality now that cost is an issue. Some of this comes out of the Total Quality Management movement initiated by W. Edwards Deming in post World War II Japan. This has been very successful in making and selling Japanese cars and televisions, but the jury is out regarding health care. TQM focuses on procedures and processes, bringing stakeholders together and utilizing brainstorming techniques to sort this all out. These procedures and processes are dissected, amplified, eliminated, changed, streamlined and substituted until customer satisfaction is achieved and resource consumption is managed. Thus, patient satisfaction is one measure of health care but, unlike the automobile industry, this can be shaky ground as the physician-patient relationship alters patient judgment. In this case the high esteem with which physicians are held by their patients often affects their assessment of clinical outcomes. Patients may put up with significant functional limitations without criticism if they have bonded with their doctor. These facts are difficult to measure; by their very nature they are obscured and kept out of view. But, during my career, I have seen it happen over and over, in different locations, circumstances, and different levels of levels of the health care experience.

So how do doctors and medical staffs deal with the quality issue? At the local level I am afraid that the effort is feeble. Most of the work done is by hospital employees who audit charts for complications and who pass on complaints. Most of the physician work is done by one or two dedicated and interested committee members, but their effort falls far short of the mark. The basis of quality management by physicians is peer review. A basic principle is that physicians have the best vantage to recognize poor quality. This presupposes that the medical staff is focused, interested, and invested in the process. Unfortunately, it does not appear to me that this is the case. In the outpatient arena, in the physician's office, the effort is even less. In community hospitals quality is a very subjective thing. It is often defined in committees as being what the most vocal, most visible, most senior, most feared, most respected, or most charismatic physician says it is. True, there is occasionally literature or experiential data to support some of these claims, but most of the time quality is not defined by science, rather, by throw weight.

Peer review is the finger in the dyke. This is where the government and people place their trust. I believe that it is often misguided trust. Peer review is an activity that all physicians are expected to participate in, but it isn't happening. At some point in the future I suspect that some outside governmental agency will gladly take over the job. This possibility falls on deaf ears. We physicians are too busy churning out procedures to be bothered. There are any number of excuses why physicians don't embrace peer review and become involved. It takes a manageable commitment each month, but it's not a popular task for several reasons; time constraints, tedium, and boredom head the list. The most ignominious objection, however, is the issue of a possible lawsuit. Peer review is a privileged endeavor. Physicians are protected from discovery when legitimately involved in the activity. There is a glitch; if restraint of trade is suspected, federal law permits discovery, sending shivers down the back of potential physician peer reviewers. Many physicians who simply opt out have cited this unlikely possibility. Even though participation is required by many medical staff bylaws, there is little will to enforce the requirement, given the threat of litigation by the threatened physician. I believe this is cowardly behavior.

Why do physicians become side tracked? The reasons are multiple. They are simply tired of study after all those years of training. They are simply too busy with the practice of medicine to have the time. What time they have left over is reserved for family affairs. Their product is "good enough" not to need much fine-tuning. They are finding it necessary to work harder, with less free time, to maintain their incomes. Deep discounts in fee for service and the ravages of capitation have had a significant pocketbook impact. None of these are good reasons. We physicians are expected to raise the bar when it comes to protecting quality. But, in the final analysis, the majority of medical staff committee time is devoted to politics, self-preservation, or mundane house keeping chores. Quality must be the centerpiece of any physician committee.

This attitude, this type of behavior, reflects basic physician flaws, which come close to the heart of the matter. Technophysicians, like myself, are so committed to preserving the status quo, their referral sources, their market share, and their affability, that they fall prey to sloppy ethics. I think that played a major role when I was doctoring Hank. If peer review is adulterated, the trickle down consequences affect the whole credentialing and privileging process, opening the door for unscrupulous physicians who have the audacity to offer procedures that they are not well trained to perform, or to offer procedures that they have not done frequently or for a long time. We come closer to understanding the nature of the health care crisis when we examine the peer review process. It is not so much the process itself, but by the players who have a vested financial interest. So, rather than throw the baby out with the wash, a better solution is to insure that our doctors are driven by some sense of ethics and morality.

Intermountain Health, headquartered in Salt Lake City, has done some good work in the quality area. This is a physician group that has taken this issue seriously and has attempted to define quality in a meaningful way. Their work has led to valuable definitions of quality and ways to hold physicians accountable. The point is made that physicians will strive harder to perform if they know that they are lagging behind their colleagues. The key is that the data, which stratifies a given group of physicians, must be anonymous. It must also be driven by science, best outcomes, and clinical guidelines. It is usually a lay person, someone familiar with statistics and clinical outcomes who does the job, and this has been one of physician's criticisms. Thus, if quality is plotted according to a personal identifying number, known only to the physician, and if a particular physician learns that his efforts are substandard, the competitive juices, which are part of the makeup of physicians, will turn on and lead to improvement. Medical education is an experience that invites each of the participants to do the best she can since it's so damn competitive. This mindset lasts a lifetime. I have been impressed with Intermountain Health's results. Physicians took the project seriously, enhanced quality, and reduced cost.

Grand Junction, Colorado has taken this one step further. This health care system makes these cost profiles, cost being an integral part of value, which also includes quality, known to all the participating physicians. This is more aggressive, putting the dirty laundry for all to see, making physicians more accountable to their peers. In one sense it is a shame to have to do this, culling out an emotion such as embarrassment to get the job done. But it works and it's simply tough shit to who disdain quality.

I must say, however, that when this stuff was tried in the hospital where I was chief of staff it fell on deaf ears. No one was interested in having an anonymous number posted for all to see. A multitude of reasons were given: the data would inevitably fall into the wrong hands, the person or persons calculating the data could not be trusted, there would be no adjustments for acuity issues, or that it wasn't necessary. Quality demands daily effort, both individually and from the corporate point of view. It is best medicine where outcomes are driven by science. Defensive medicine is inappropriate. Self-serving behavior is anathema. Ignorance is no excuse. Physicians need to look to quality studies that help define clinical outcomes, which in turn helps the physician choose the best diagnostic or therapeutic option.

So, what is quality. I have outlined different takes on quality, but I have a slightly different slant, born from the tragedy of Hank. It is woven within the Hippocratic Oath. It is part of the vocation or calling of being a doctor. I believe that it has to be seen within the definition of value. Whatever definition of quality is accepted, physicians must be good stewards, conscious of the costs attendant to a diagnostic or therapeutic decisions. Clinical outcomes must be born from the scientific method. But, here is the difference; this information must by leavened by spiritual considerations. As I have already said, I believe that allopathic medicine by itself has come up short when dealing with chronic disease. Thus, this is a major challenge for today's physicians as medical education is focused upon reductionist methodology. But, again it hasn't been effective with chronic disease and I don't believe it will be. Of course, physicians must commit to regular reading, attending medical conferences, and participating in local medical meetings. I believe in board certification and recertification. We must practice within the confines of our specialty, not venturing outside to increase our incomes. But, we must also include the metaphysical elements of healing, which presupposes a new type of learning. Quality will be well served when this happens. I will have more to say about that. In the final analysis, there must be some way to document our individual effort and this information must be made public. There actually may be a role for the AMA here, to insist that physicians commit to this task, and where public opinion has a role to play.

And so it is. Quality is often just given lip service. Value is obscured. Hospital administration sees quality as holding down costs and not having too many medical misadventures without much attention to the overall value of the procedure. There is some data which attests to better results for complicated procedures at high volume centers, but this is often disdained by physicians in smaller community hospitals who respond with the notion that they were trained to do said procedure and they don't need any help. And, because of the resiliency of Homo sapiens, ala Evans, they often get away with predictable complications. Patients are not privy to any of this and if they were it might not make much difference, since they have bonded with their physicians. We now have a new health care reality in part driven by a commendable intent to provide insurance to the most vulnerable amongst us, but the weakest link will be quality.

As the government becomes more involved it will have the authority to define quality with the focus mostly upon cost and availability. After all, the government will hold the purse strings. I believe that this most certainly will happen. Rest assured, when the government becomes involved in a financial partnership, it plays its trump card with the purse strings. Perhaps something is better than nothing, but we shouldn't accept anything less than the best. And the best is a physician community that makes quality a number one consideration, without governmental coercion. Since physicians are well positioned to measure and define quality, our efforts must be directed towards them, ensuring that they take this job seriously, that their attitudes change, that moral and ethical elements are infused into the process. If that doesn't happen, then they do not deserve to be the quality makers. I will have more to say about how this could happen.

Chapter 8
Technophysicians: Where Trust Is Lost

The years of private practice provided additional illumination, bringing into focus a dysfunctional health care system, a patois of high technology, managed care, complimentary care, uncompensated care and government intervention. The fabric of health care was beginning to be torn, frayed, and weakened, anything but seamless. Physicians began to act out. They were heard to bitterly complain and to leave asunder the service aspects of doctoring because of discounted fees for service, managed care, insensitive bureaucrats, ambivalent hospital administrators, and non-compliant patients. A fault line developed between cognitive physicians, i.e. internists, pediatricians, family physicians, general practitioners, and the higher paid technophysicians, i.e. surgeons, cardiologists, nephrologists, and gastroenterologists. These were years characterized by more and more big brother, physicians leaving practice, and the growth of IPA, PPOs, and HMOs, a veritable smorgasbord of payment schemes, all designed to hold down costs, decimate quality, and ensure healthy profits for the health care engineers. More and more private physicians were joining mega groups. Fewer physicians were participating in hospital affairs. Technophysicians were demanding that the hospital pay for their after hour services. More and more uninsured were using the ER for routine illnesses. Fewer technophysicians were providing backup call for the ER. Health care became a juggernaut, hurling into anarchy, rudderless, a theater for the disaffected and disillusioned.

What I learned from Hank, namely the importance of what I had learned from the interaction between Dr. Fontaine and Mary Little, was neatly tucked away in my brain, a guidepost of sorts, but not an active part of thinking. My own journey had led me to physician leadership positions, culminating in being elected simultaneously as chief of staff of two hospitals about to merge. The merger of these hospitals was a study of Machiavellian intrigue. Orchestrating the merged medical staff, with all its attendant officers, committees, and subcommittees, left me with any number of arrows in my back. I became an easy target, as physicians needed some tangible human being to attack. There were some victories, but at great price. Disgruntled physicians acted out by jumping onto the due process wagon whenever there was a perceived injustice. Perceived injustices ranged from simple criticism to restriction of privileges. It was with these events as a background that I came to understand more about the root causes of this fragmenting health care system

I became part of a process for hospital redesign, an effort to streamline access and flow, injecting multitasking, a trial of electronic medical records, and the invitation for physicians to carefully consider continuous quality improvement. Change is often anathema, a threat to stability, and health care is no exception.

Paradoxically, at the same time, I was becoming more and more of a technophysician. All of my training subsequently coalesced into something quite different than I first imagined. In spite of Hank and Mary Little, the years of specialty training had stripped me of notions of holism and healing. Those aspects of health care seemed irrelevant and unnecessary. I measured my competence by recording the number of advanced procedures I had accomplished, the bravado attendant to making procedure related decisions, and the approval I received from my mentors and colleagues. I had much to learn, yet I was now an anointed member of that fraternity of physicians trained to embrace high technology, trained to strip the magic of health care to its basics, impatient with Dr. Fontaine's tools, and prepared to dive into the restoration of disordered pathophysiology with fancy gadgets. This created inner tension, something that fosters growth, but certainly not a comfortable state of mind.

Let's talk a little bit more about technophysicians. I am not talking about technomedicine, which has given us marvelous tools for health care. I am talking about we physicians who grab hold of one the rings on the technomedicine merry-go-round and trade our particular device or gimmick for greed, avarice, control; anything but healing. Technophysicians gravitate towards technomedicine much like a magnet. This unsavory bonding between the two is a cause for concern. This symbiosis is at the heart of attitudes which germinate in training and permeate the industry, and leave in its wake the notion that anything goes at the risk of subordinating healing to successfully carrying out a procedure. This attitude affects many layers of the health care team, but most especially primary care physicians who come to believe that engaging this bonded entity is the accepted norm, leaving aside their own take of a particular problem. Healing is stuck at the gate without a chance to play a meaningful role. I know what I am talking about since I had become a technophysician.

****

During the first 50 years of the 20th century American medicine became the standard bearer for the rest of the world. American medical schools have produced the finest doctors, American medical research has been the envy of the world, and as a result, infectious diseases and nutritional deficiency diseases have nearly been put to rest. As an outgrowth of World War II, research has led to marvelous ways for dealing with trauma and deprivation. There was every reason in the world for an individual to put his or her faith and trust in our doctors and their ministrations given these marvelous victories. After World War II a technological explosion occurred, a direct consequence of the ascendancy of American medical research, with a profound impact on health care.

This technology arose in tertiary, academic medical centers and developed with the imprint of the scientific method. In the beginning, scientific inquiry and the technological outgrowth were closely aligned and qualified as applied science. Unseen at the time, however, was a subtle bifurcation of science and technology. Slowly and surely, the technological fruit of scientific research became a force unto itself, foisted on patients by technophysicians, demanding veneration, which rightly belonged to the scientists. Technomedicine, a profitable outgrowth of science, now masquerading as science, was sold to patients by technophysicians, and has continued to be the recipient of this seductive relationship. The positive results claimed by science has obfuscated the profits and mischief created by many technophysicians.

Science was king following World War II. The federal government loosened its purse strings, providing a plethora of funds to medical researchers for any number of projects, some good, and some bad. The traditional balance of the medical school mission subtly shifted from patient care and education, to research. This was the golden era of medical science and technology.

Specialty physicians who have become technophysicians, an inevitable outgrowth of the bifurcation of science and technology, and hospitals have joined an unhealthy alliance during the past generation. Specialty physicians, who had a gimmick to sell, and whom I have defined as technophysicians, found that the community hospital was a ready and willing partner. Well-trained physicians, who might otherwise become faculty, loosened their relationships with academic health care centers and jumped into the community hospital arena. Why not? The hospitals were looking for an edge, an increased market share, profitability and stature. With the proper support, these technophysicians could do as good a job in a community hospital as in a teaching hospital and in the community hospital there is more freedom, less academic baggage, and lots of money. It was a win win situation.

With a snap of the finger, the ethical and scientific justification to do procedures was subordinated to less savory motivations: greed, control, power, and self-gratification. The decision to place a feeding tube, an invasive surgical procedure, in a dying patient locked in a futile battle, is more attuned to personal gain than help for the patient. The decision to keep a terminally ill patient in the ICU has very little to do with the proper use of technology. The decision to remove a gall bladder from a demented, frail patient with congestive heart failure when the indication is simply gall stones incidentally noted on an ultrasound, is obscene at best. This sad state of affairs dispels the notion that technmedicine is a branch of science or that the two are the same. Technomedicine has become a methodology whereby unscrupulous doctors bastardize science in an effort to promote their own agenda. No one is able to oversee the operation since the new technophysicians are so highly trained, above scrutiny, and well connected with the university. Specialist physicians, those highly trained specialists with a commitment to the proper use of high technology, were in demand, coveted by hospitals and patients, both of whom had confidence in the scientific validity of invasive and intrusive testing. This, of course, was entirely appropriate. But when avarice replaces altruism, when some specialist physicians morphed into technophysicians, the clinical indications were attenuated such that simply having an available orifice was good enough for some gastroenterologists. The result, I believe, is that these technophysicians are responsible for much of the rising health care expenditures. We technophysicians have put ourselves in a position to determine the demand for our own services. We are the ones who drive the machine. Add to all of that the notion sold to all of us that advances in modern medicine will probably lead to immortality, a disease-free existence, and it is not hard to fathom why we technophysicians have had our way. What family would decline to sign a consent for a procedure recommended by a technophysician when told that their loved one is likely to die if it is not done. At times this is true. But a bone fide specialty physician would explain the pros and cons, offering alternatives that do not necessarily include technology, willing to stay involved even if his role is simply supportive. Not so with technophysicians who simply schedule a procedure.

At the same time we technophysicians have turned away from any need to show compassion and caring for the patient. We weave our magic isolated from patient, removed from the messy reality of suffering, comforted by the detachment provided by machines, lenses, screens, and anesthesia. When I first landed in Sacramento I worked in a multispecialty group that included an interesting hematologist/oncologist. He was a very smart guy, imposing in stature, and very up to date. On more than one occasion I watched him make rounds in the hospital. Much as we did in Los Angeles County General Hospital, he piled the metal charts in a grocery cart and with a nurse at his side simply talked to whatever patient, but from the doorway. He never actually entered the room, never touched the patient, never looked him in the eyes, and gave perfunctory answers to the frightened patient's questions. He maintained this calculated distance from the patient, perhaps to protect his own soul, or maybe he didn't like his job.

My brother was an F-4 fighter pilot during the Vietnam War. He related to me the detachment he felt, his body insulated and wrapped with sophisticated machinery, racing across the sky, which obscured the carnage he caused below when bombs were dropped. It is much the same with technophysicians. The ministrations of technophysicians, whether good or bad, are separated, as it were, not a part of any intimate experience, simply events recorded by computers, seen through lenses and video screens.

Obviously there are fine physicians who use technology appropriately and are a credit to the profession. Unfortunately, there are enough unscrupulous technophysicians who use technomedicine for their own selfish benefit, driving up the cost of health care. If health care costs are now three trillion dollars a year, I would estimate that one third of this number is due to the inappropriate use of high technology. I have come to believe that this is where we need to focus our attention, not in finding ways to underwrite the costs attributable to these charlatans. This is in essence what was accomplished with the recent passage of the Obama health care reform. I don't believe that the politicians who pushed this legislation are malicious. They are on the one hand misinformed, and on the other anxious to claim approval for fixing the health care malfunction. This they did not do. Universal access to quality medicine is the goal, which no governmental financial scheme can promise to provide. Self-serving technophysicians are where the spotlight belongs, and this has to change. Focusing on systems alone is missing the point. The audacity with which technophysicians approach health care is breathtaking. For we technophysicians, decisions to use technology have had more to do with pocket book issues than quality.

We technophysicians are willing to try out a new technique, having been given the briefest of instruction by a manufacturing representative and having had little or no experience with actually doing the procedure. We technophysicians are convinced that our training and experience preclude any careful mastery of a new procedure. Even if this new procedure is simply a modification of an existing one, patients who put themselves into the hands of technophysicians, are handing over trust, which is at best is unearned, finding themselves in harm's way. Technophysicians simply take advantage of the situation. Case selection becomes subordinated to one of the two axioms Evans taught me: that 95% of patients will get well regardless of what is done to them, and families want everything done during the last 6 months of life. These two axioms are invitations for misbehavior, mischief, and mistakes, especially if they are simply a justification to do procedures. This is convenient for we technophysicians.

The process of becoming or the pathway to healing is a powerful force. I've had to learn this the hard way. The tragedy of Hank is imbedded in my soul. Healing is appropriate for all illnesses, even those that are easily cured with antibiotics. Illness affects all of us is subtle ways apart from the success of curing. When we are sick, even with the simplest of afflictions, our take of ourselves, our sense of mortality, our adjustment to our environment, are all called into question. The patients that I have seen during my 40 years of practice all have questions about their lives, their behavior, and their relationships. These questions may be hidden, but the careful practitioner will provide am opportunity for these questions. Many doctors will tell you that they don't have time for these questions, but patients don't take much time to ask and share their concerns. I am happy to have finally learned this.

The trappings of today's hospital health care delivery system has changed and is changing, an effort to hold down costs without much regard to quality. No longer does the private physician admit and care for a patent when hospitalization is needed. In fact, the so-called personal physician often sends patients to the ER for a determination if hospitalization is needed. This has become the norm during the past ten years. Hospitalists are doctors employed by the hospital to manage the care of inpatients. The task of throwing the patient to the wolves, to shiny citadels of healing, is left to an overworked, fatigued, and harried ER doctor, who often has an attitude because of the stream of underserved patients who are searching for relief and assistance. The ER doctor deftly hands off the patient to a hospitalist who is in the pocket of the technophysician. So the unwary patient becomes cannon fodder for the next layer, which often includes a technophysician who promises depersonalization and dangerous tests. The captain of the team, who was formerly the patient's private physician, is now an amorphous entity, whatever hospitalist happens to be on call, and often only a task oriented person. No one is around to coordinate the in- patient experience, no one other than the social worker, who may or may not understand the nature of the problem.

So how does this happen? How does the hospital's organized medical staff grant privileges to physicians who need to be approved as a member of the active medical staff in order to ply their craft. The process allows unscrupulous individuals to become prosperous technophysicians? The state and federal government have given physicians the authority to ensure that physicians who practice in the hospital are well trained, not only in the technical aspects of a procedure, but also possessing the knowledge when to apply the technology, and how to integrate the potential results of the procedure within the context of the patient's total care. This is huge discretionary power, which is often treated in a cavalier way.

This process is called credentialing, a place where the public entrusts physicians to ensure that a candidate is up to snuff. Credentialing is the time-honored process by which a hospital medical staff satisfies itself that a particular physician has been properly trained, who he says he is, namely a graduate of an accredited medical school, someone who has successfully completed a post graduate training program, who is able to perform at a level equal to or better than others within the same specialty. The hospital Board of Trustees assumes that this administrative process is done well by the medical staff since there is much legal exposure. If a physician makes it through this process, he is cleared to practice his specialty and perform those procedures integral to his specialty forever, whether or not he does it frequently, whether or not he keeps his skills in intact, whether or not he has even done the procedure since his training days. A reapplication request is simply rubber-stamped. This is slowly changing (slowly is the operative word), but asking physicians to provide a glimpse of their current experience with a particular procedure is like pulling hen's teeth. Medical staff bylaws protect the physician. Since he was successful with his original credentialing effort, the board of trustees, the hospital, and the medical staff assume it is his inalienable right granted for perpetuity. If a physician requests a new procedure and persuades the credentials committee that it is simply a modification of an existing procedure, credentialing is usually granted without much sweat.

Again and again physicians are cavalierly granted high-tech privileges. New physicians right out of a training program are usually up to date and highly skilled with the latest in their fields. The medical staff comforts itself with the list of successfully completed procedures, communication with his/her mentors, and a proctoring process. Most of this is casually done, without much effort in communicating with the applicant's mentors. In fact, many times the task of authenticating the application of new physicians is assumed by the medical staff secretary and signed off by the chief of staff. In many instances there is a "good old boy" mentality. If the prospective applicant trained at a well-known institution scrutiny is attenuated. If someone on the medical staff credentials committee personally knows the applicant, or one of his mentors, the guy's in. If an applicant is really bad, if he has had a number of malpractice events, if adverse information precedes his appearance before the committee, if there is a subtle bias about his style of medicine, privileges may not be granted. This doesn't happen often and when it does the applicant physician often becomes litigious, engaging the medical staff and the board of trustees in a nasty legal battle. The law supports a properly done credentialing process, but physician leaders often succumb to the threatening rhetoric of the disgruntled physician and his council. There is not much interest in confronting a colleague.

Applying a meaningful credentialing process or ensuring that the physician is qualified, is a bigger problem with physicians who have been out of training for awhile and who want to get involved with these new sexy procedures. When the procedure or operation is simply a minor modification of a more basic procedure, it is less of an issue. When the high tech endeavor is something radically new, physicians are very generous to one another. There are issues of financial reward and turf protection. The medical staff could require more but that rarely occurs. This scenario is virtually the same with any specialty. Rarely is there much of a requirement to learn a procedure as well as had been done during the residency years.

Carrying out new procedures or operations thus become on the job training, often learned from sales persons, and complications are many times deftly swept under the rug. If a delicate and complicated procedure learned by a physician many years ago is the issue, and if the physician has rarely done the procedure in later years, this is a major issue if the physician wants to do the procedure. The organized medical staff rarely has the courage to require a brush up course or ensure that someone else does the job or helps out. Doctors learn how to do the job of doctoring in their training years, yet their proficiency falls off when they don't do a procedure frequently. In a life saving situation the stakes are different. But in an elective situation where their skills are not up to par, patients find themselves in the cross hairs of danger because the medical staff does not step in. The problem arises when the physician in question does the procedure anyway, motivated by something other than quality, subordinating the patient's best interests to a less savory motive. There are many doctors who's training is suspect, whose skills are rusty, or who have never properly learned new techniques since graduating. This is not information that we patients are privy to. We assume that when someone is called a specialist, when there are diplomas on the wall attesting to that fact, when the doctor in question has been around for some time and is known by many in the medical community, that we are safer. The fact is that we are not safer; not safer unless we are assured that our doctor's training is firm, that he is up to date and performs whatever procedure frequently without complications, that he took the requisite time and training to improve his skills and learn new techniques, and his decision to act is predicated on a thorough evaluation of the patient. All of this is assumed or taken for granted when we establish a covenant with the specialist to whom we have been referred. The message is to be wary, to require that our specialist earns our trust, that we are confident that this person is up to date, has been doing whatever procedure frequently, and has a good track record.

Mistakes are inevitably made when inadequately trained physicians are involved. Yet, all too often these physicians have been granted privileges by the medical staff. When I came to Maui to practice I learned that general surgeons were doing much of the colonoscopy because there was a dearth of properly trained gastroenterologists. I have nothing against surgeons doing colonoscopy if they have been properly trained. This is not always the case, and a shortage of trained physicians is no excuse for allowing poorly trained surgeons fill the gap. But it has happened and recently a healthy man suffered a bowel perforation when a poorly trained surgeon submitted a patient to colonoscopy. The patient died and this may lead to a malpractice event. However, there has been no effort by the local medical staff to deal with the basic issue, namely that poorly prepared individuals are being granted privileges for whatever reason. This happens everywhere. This is not to say that complications do not occur even in the hands of properly trained physicians. They certainly do, but at a much lower rate.

This begs the question of how to insure that there is not a shortage of well trained physicians. This may become an issue if we citizens insist that our physicians are well equipped with proper training and ethical ballast. If the number of technophysicians falls and the number of properly trained specialists increases, then there should be no problem. Well trained specialty physicians should be well paid, but only if they can demonstrate to our satisfaction that they have not only the requisite technical skills, but a sense of propriety, honestly about their abilities, and an attitude that the practice of medicine is a vocation and not just a job. This assumes that physician leaders take seriously the task of the credentialing process. I believe that this task will inevitably fall to physicians, since physicians understand this stuff, but physicians who themselves have ethical underpinnings. It may be worthwhile considering a system whereby lay persons would participate in the credentialing process. This would be anathema to physicians, but it might improve the process.

How can this happen? Aren't there regulatory agencies that supervise the process? Doesn't the government have a stake in the process? The answer is yes and no. The Joint Commission of Accredited Hospitals has been given the statutory authority to oversee this process. The joint commission is a group of senior physicians, nurses, and other health care persons, usually retired and supplementing their retirement, who may or may not have a clue about quality health care. Their mandate is to insure that the medical staff is faithful to their own bylaws. This is a fairly superficial task that is tediously carried out, but with little inclination to tear asunder the medical staff bylaws or to carefully assess quality. The rub is that the medical staff bylaws are often a product of technophysicians and their friends. It is as good and faithful to quality as the physicians who craft the bylaws make it. The general medical staff is often a group of uninterested physicians who rarely attend general medical staff meetings, and rarely attend committees and subcommittees to which they are assigned. They usually support what the Medical Executive Committee presents to them. While the MEC could demand more effort from the credentialing committee, technophysicians are often embedded in the MEC, carefully orchestrating an outcome that is favorable to them.

Shouldn't the government become more involved? The answer is again yes and no. I believe that physicians are best position to define quality. Political leaders, scientists, and concerned citizens are at a disadvantage as they are not calling the shots. Medicine has for years been a closed shop. The substance of medical education is not privy to lay persons. This is so in part to protect the integrity of medicine, to regulate physician membership, to safeguard physician remuneration, and to represent parochial medical issues with a single voice. But this situation is often abused, providing a safe haven for unscrupulous physicians who make up the rank of technophysicians, leaving the profession and public in a quandary. So, we are left with the notion that only physicians can define and regulate quality, yet the definition of quality can be adulterated by technophysicians who can lower the bar for whatever reason. The issue of quality is subtle, wrapped within the layers of medical education, constantly changing by the nuances of scientific advancement. To stay involved takes work; work done by well educated physicians, who are involved in the practice of medicine, who are motivated by a commitment to best practice. Lay individuals could participate. I believe that they would recognize the properly trained physician and provide oversight and support the proper process of credentialing and the granting of privileges.

How can we recognize a technophysician? He or she is usually in a hurry, unable to sit quietly and listen to the story that patients yearn to tell their doctor. There is little eye contact, the physician wears a visage of impatience, marginal physical contact exists between the doctor and patient, and a cursory physical examination takes place. The time honored history taking and physical examination skills have been subordinated to imposing machines, with computer printouts, flashing lights, and intimidating sounds. The stethoscope, ophthalmoscope, sphigmomoneter, reflex hammer have all been relegated to the dump heap, a reminder of the fate of my black bag. There is a rush to schedule whatever procedure the technophysician is selling, with a perfunctory explanation, and hurried informed consent. This scenario may be different under different circumstances, but the elements of haste, indifference, and a rush to high technology, without a proper explanation, are common to technophysicians.

In my experience patients intuitively recognize these base elements, which are the foundation of their discomfort.

Why do we let technophysicians do this? Because we can get away with it. The system has blessed us with a carte blanche, a not-so benevolent approval, and patients have cosigned the whole thing. Do we technophysicians do these things because we actually believe that the outcomes justify the ordeal? Sometimes, but more often than not, there are other perfidious motivations at work. The system itself is calcified, unable to remold itself, satisfied that high technology is inherently the right answer. The medical educational system invites students to follow without question the advice and recommendations of teachers, instilling a herd mentality, and leaving the spawning technophysician with precious little objectivity in deciding who should or should not have a procedure. This coupled with the monetary rewards paves the way for unscrupulous technophysicians who are busy contributing mightily to the ever-increasing rise in health care expenditures.

****

On a rainy Sunday afternoon I was asked to see a patient in consultation that had just had coronary bypass surgery. Postoperatively, the patient developed abdominal distention, fever, and tenderness. The possible diagnoses ranged from a ruptured internal organ with peritonitis to a vascular accident resulting in poor blood supply to the intestines, leading to gangrene. Either of these could be fatal, and not at all what the cardiac surgeon had in mind. Cardiac surgeons want few complications on their dossier. If there are coexisting medical issues, if the patient has other co-morbidities, the wise surgeon will ask an internal medical consultant to be involved.

One of the first jobs of the consultant is to review the entire chart, the old history, interview the nurses, review the x-rays, and come to some sort of conclusion. Patients undergo procedures for specific reasons. In this case unstable angina, or an impending myocardial infarct was the reason. Whatever the indication, there must be a reasonable expectation that the patient will be better off with the procedure. In other words, the risk of doing the procedure should be significantly outweighed by the benefit expected. But, it takes more than a reason to subject a patient to a complicated and delicate procedure. The patient must want it, or if he is unable to communicate, there should be some acknowledged indication that the effort would be approved. He must be reasonably stable. In an emergency this is not relevant, but with semi-elective, or elective surgery, the patient's general condition should be conducive. The risk benefit ratio should clearly favor doing the procedure; not just successfully completing the procedure; the patient should be the recipient of quality, enjoying a return of function, not simply vegetating with a repaired organ.

There should be no absolute contraindications. If the patient is feeble and fragile, and a procedure carries an unacceptably high mortality, it should not be done. If the patient has another co morbid condition, and already is wrestling with a futile situation, then the wise surgeon will pass on the procedure. Absolute contraindications include coexisting terminal cancer, multiple uncontrolled co morbidities, a severe infection in some other part of the body, or "Do Not Resuscitate" wish on the chart.

Relative contraindications are treated differently. These range from impaired renal function to age, but as indicated above, when taken together they may point to a more conservative approach.

This particular patient was a Jehovah's Witness with chronic renal failure, a significant anemia, and in her eighties. Do any of these preclude bypass surgery? Not necessarily, but in the aggregate the decision to operate was highly questionable. Bypass surgery is very difficult, fraught with potential complications, not the least of which is untoward bleeding. A JW patient, citing scriptural justification in the Old Testament, is adamantly opposed to receiving blood or blood products. There are hospitals, which deal with this issue, using plasma expanders, but not blood products, and they do a fairly good job at managing this situation. However, we were not in that type of hospital, nor was any effort made to arrange for this. The decision was made to operate given the additional risk, which was buried in the arcane verbiage of the informed consent.

This lady had significant kidney failure from chronic hypertension. She was not uremic, nor in need of dialysis, but her kidneys were working over time to clear waste products and keep the ship of state afloat. Does renal failure preclude cardiac surgery? Not always. However, her renal function was so precarious preoperatively that complete shutdown was a possibility. Yet, the decision was made to operate.

She had a significant anemia. Her hemoglobin was less than sufficient to effectively carry oxygen to her tissues. Patients usually adjust to chronic anemia with compensatory shifts in the oxygen dissociation curve facilitating the release of oxygen from hemoglobin, the molecules that are within red blood cells and that bind to and carry this oxygen to our tissues. Would an anemia preclude taking a patient to surgery for a coronary bypass? No, especially not if we could plan on a transfusion. Sometimes delicate procedures are done because of an ongoing anemia. But, as indicated above, this was a chronic anemia and a transfusion out of the question.

Finally, she was in her eighties. Do we deny patients life-saving procedures because of age? Certainly not. At the same time common sense is needed. It is not simply an issue of prolonging a patient's life, but rather, improving the quality of that life. Hence, in elderly patients, without a DNR, the reasonable approach would be to include the patient, or the surrogate, in a discussion regarding outcomes, complications, and future quality of life. None of this of course happened. There was a brief informed consent discussion with this frail, sick, and elderly woman. These discussions are often cursory, loaded with complicated words, with the emphasis on the dire consequences if the procedure is not completed. I learned much of this from her nurse who was present during the so-called informed consent. This is the way it often goes. The patient and the family are so impressed with the trappings of high tech medicine, so trusting of the doctors, understandably wanting everything done, but left naïve about the hard cold facts. Nurses, clergy, and social workers are rarely invited to participate in the informed consent discussion. The hospital has a proprietary right to have some sort of form signed by the patient and a witness attesting to acknowledging informed consent. This is casually done by the technophysician after what passes for informed consent, without much regard to meaningful informed consent. The admonition regarding the last 6 months of life becomes operative and so the drama unfolds.

The decision to operate is owned by the cardiac surgeon, a huge conflict of interest. He has a supporting cast of cardiologists, primary care physicians, the patient's family and, of course, the patient if he is able; but not infrequently these individuals are pressed into giving their blessing, given the "dire consequences" presented by the technophysician. This is the case with any technophysician. They are the darlings of the health care industry, accounting for a significant amount of the hospital's revenue stream, glorified by the press, actually coming to believe that they are something special.

This JW patient who was operated on did suffer a vascular accident to the small bowel because of preexisting mesenteric atherosclerosis and a period of diminished perfusion pressure. She underwent another emergency operation where nearly all of her small bowel was found to be ischemic, infarcted, and gangrenous because of inadequate blood flow and oxygen. This is incompatible with life and the patient ultimately died.

So it is with we technophysicians. To be first on the block is heady tonic. To be a leader is intoxicating. Power and control are powerful energizers, not to mention financial success. Doctoring is something quite different. It presupposes that the physician includes healing along with curing; healing, that intangible life force which derives from feeling, caring, empathy, altruism, and intuition. Hope is an integral part of healing. I have seen patients with incurable cancer who were unresponsive to conventional therapy, survive and live many more productive years than expected, simply with hope. This is what is missing. The healing aspects of medicine are left wanting, not part of the technophysician's agenda, and too time consuming.

****

The decision to treat a terminal patient with chemotherapy represents a sad and unhappy situation. There have been many victories by oncologists, not the least being the successful treatment of childhood leukemias. Other regimens have given added quality of life to cancer sufferers. My own opinion is that physicians will look back at this approach to malignancies much as we regard alchemy. Giving toxic chemicals, which invariably destroy normal tissue, in an effort to slow or halt the spread of cancer, is at best a hit and miss proposition. The hope and expectation is that the malignant cells will be destroyed at a faster rate than normal cells, so that there is a viable human organism after the ordeal. The side effects are devastating. Invariably, those normal cells in our bodies, which divide more frequently than others, are affected, because chemotherapeutic agents confuse them with malignant cells. Today new therapies target molecules integral to the survival of these rapidly dividing cancer cells adding a new dimension to cancer treatment. These new drugs are antibodies to cytokines, the messengers that pave the way for cancer cell expansion, and outcomes have improved. But, all of this has a profound effect on a cancer patient's quality of life, that precious time left before death.

The problem is that the structure of the reimbursement system for doctors who treat patients with metastatic cancer has in the past created a financial conflict of interest that had a powerful influence on the physician and the potential for harm for these vulnerable patients.

The decision to treat is often simply to assuage the family or to offer a glimmer of hope in an otherwise futile situation. That is not necessarily a bad thing. Hope is a powerful tool and I have seen many patients with lethal tumors survive for many years where hope was the main therapeutic agent. Not infrequently, I am asked to search for the primary, the organ and tissue from whence the cancer sprung, ostensibly to help the oncologist choose a chemotherapy program. If the cancer is wide spread, involving multiple organs, then I am not certain I see the point of subjecting a very sick patient to a number of intrusive tests. But I have done it, more motivated by financial rewards, than altruism. For me, at least, the path of proper medical ethics was blurred by behavior that substituted expediency for propriety. This behavior grew from my experiences in medical school, residency, and private practice, where I learned to subordinate healing to curing. In my experience the commitment to curing is more costly because of increased dividends for the technophysician and the hospital. This often adds unnecessary costs and suffering with very little expectation that there will be a significant improvement in the patient's situation. To my surprise, I have found that offering hope in a futile situation is efficacious, less dangerous, and much less expensive. The trick is to understand when a patient's condition is futile, where dangerous drugs will only add to the patient's misery, and when spiritual tools are more appropriate. I will have more to say about spiritual tools, but it is incumbent for the specialty physician, as well as the attending clinician, to clearly understand when the situation is futile, an understanding that comes with proper medical education, an understanding that must not be dismissed because there is an opportunity to integrate a lucrative, but ineffectual, procedure in the dying patient's care plan.

    I recently saw a 41-year-old mother of two in consultation. She was initially referred with abdominal pain and abnormal liver function tests. Imaging studies were highly suspicious for metastatic cancer to the liver. A biopsy of the liver confirmed this impression. The tissue type was adenocarcinoma, cells that had originally arisen from some solid organ somewhere else in the body. The presupposition was that if the primary could be ascertained, there was a better chance for response. That is the key word— response. In some instances, if the primary were colon cancer, there is some hope for prolonging meaningful life, but not much. Otherwise, the outlook is gloomy. She was admitted to the hospital with some neurological symptoms and was unfortunately found to have brain involvement. This did respond to the temporary palliative affect of irradiation, but this complication further portended a very gloomy prognosis. Because of this desperate situation, I got off the hook and didn't feel pressured to search for the primary.

The real issue for the patient was whether the additional benefit of chemotherapy, namely prolonging life, was worth it; would this be quality time, without pain, with mental clarity, with some hope that she could enjoy the remaining time with her husband and children? She honestly wrestled with this issue. Her family was supportive, helping her see the pros and cons, not caught up in the hysteria of the moment, needing information from the oncologist which was not readily forthcoming. Being an oncologist is a very difficult task. It is much easier to say that there is a treatment, and that the situation appears to be more futile without chemotherapy. Some of this attitude is genuine, but many times cavalier at best. There is clearly a payoff for enrolling the patient in a chemotherapeutic treatment plan. Until recently there was a glitch here, a gimmick for oncologists. Oncologists learned that it was legal to purchase intravenous medications at wholesale and charge the patient a hefty price at the retail level. Outpatient chemotherapy with parenteral chemotherapeutic agents thus became very profitable. CMS has stepped in put a halt to this, but until recently this conflict of interest was at the heart of decisions made to administer chemotherapy. Oral chemotherapeutic agents continue to be bought and sold in the doctors office. Oncologists buy drugs from wholesalers, mark them up and sell them to patients in the office. Gatesman and Smith write in the November 3, 2011 New England of Medicine that "since medical oncology is a cognitive specialty lacking associated procedures, without drug sales, oncologists' salaries would be lower than geriatricians". In other words, since oncologists do not have a gimmick, they have found a favorable business model. I believe that a lack of moral ballast has adulterated the focus at the point of service in this situation, as it does in many other situations where the opportunity to do a procedure or operate is approved by all, including the patient and family, because "something is being done." Doing "something" is a bill of goods that organized medicine has sold to the public in spite of the fact that the likelihood of success is slim to none. Doing "something" has obscured the more base motivation of personal gain, a convenient situation for the technophysician. I was once told by a seasoned professor, when confronted with a futile situation, to "don't just do something, stand there." That seems a bit insensitive, but makes the point that we physicians are not in control, that there is an answer that derives from a higher power, that is often neglicted and under utilized.

We technophysicians face a major conflict when deciding to perform a procedure or operation. We are trained to intervene. We are trained to be bold, making a firm decision, not to equivocate. Only infrequently does a technophysician decline to become involved. The issues of money, control, and reputation are powerful and are woven within the tapestry of this decision. It is very difficult for a technophysician to pass on a procedure, which he/she is good at performing, and which promises rewards. It is especially difficult when patients so readily acquiesce, asking few if any questions, not demanding important information, which helps make an informed decision. Trusting patients behave like sheep, blindly following the holy grail of high tech medicine, blinded by the sexy technology, over-awed by those physicians we have made larger than life.

The point of all of this is that without the underpinning of honesty, and proper credentialing, issues like case selection will inevitably be relegated to the scrap heap of duplicity. Technophysicians will be encouraged to "do something." Health care expenditures will continue to rise until, or unless, the government steps in with draconian measures that will indiscriminately ration care by fiat, which will adversely affect both physicians and patients, or until patients insist on a better effort by their doctors. It is more than just the quality issues of credentialing, training, and experience. The process of credentialing and granting privileges is more than ensuring that the applicant physician has successfully competed the requisite training and possesses the required skills. The intangible element of physician judgment needs to be examined. An examination of these intangible elements is difficult, but medical staffs need to develop methodologies to do the job. Thus, the medical staff credentialing committee may need to have lay membership, individuals with expertise in these issues, perhaps clergy, psychologists, retired physicians, or seasoned nurses. These are moral/ethical issues, which are usually ignored or passed over casually. But they are essential and we citizens need to be confident that our specialist has passed this muster, that he understands the spiritual side of the equation. This is an area that is woefully shortchanged. The self-serving decision to use technology for profit becomes a moral dilemma. Technology used inappropriately can be deadly. The customer, or patients, often has insufficient information to make an independent choice. Medical information has been so controlled by organized medicine that few patients have access to this data to help them make an independent evaluation. Customers, who are all of us, need to be confident that our specialist physician has moral ballast, a spiritual connection of some sorts, and the intangible skills of empathy and intuition.

The sad fact is that there is precious little evidence that our technophysicians have moral ballast. The best evidence, or lack of, comes from nurses who work in hospitals, especially acute care units. These individuals see up front and personal the jump to high technology in futile situations, when less invasive approaches are treated with disdain, and when patients are left without proper information and compassion. The first task is to understand that this is so, that more often than not, we find ourselves in harms way when we are treated by a technophysician. We can count on the resilience of Homo sapiens to bail us out, but there are times when our luck runs out.

In the next two chapters we will explore how the two neglected stepchildren of the technophysician-technomedicine bond suffer. Continuing education and professionalism are causalities of this bond, and their demise is a certainty with either the status quo or government medicine. I have watched with dismay the disintegration of these stepchildren. My own experiences referenced above, added clarity to my observations, which portends the end of American medicine, as we know it, unless something is done. These next two chapters characterize the epicenters of dysfunction, the results of spiritually bankrupt medicine, and hopefully leading to a wakeup call for us all.

Chapter 9
THE PINK SLIP: Continuing Education—An Afterthought

Continuing medical education, which is fundamental to the practice of good medicine, is mostly a burden to technophysicians. CME is a requirement by regulatory agencies and the government to ensure physician commitment, but in the final analysis meaningless for technophysicians who treat CME with the same passion as renewing a drivers license. For the most part it is seen as a burden and the easiest way to get it done is the best.

Most of the states have requirements, which expect a physician to "earn" so many hours of continuing education as a requisite for maintaining or issuing a license. Aside from the fact that these audits are infrequent and rarely enforced, there is a fundamental nonchalant attitude on the part of technophysicians. They get the hours because that is the requirement, but there is very little learning or retention of material that would be helpful in their individual practices or in the struggle to stay involved with quality. What actually passes for CME includes boondoggle trips to exotic places, credits "earned" by signing in at hospital conferences that have little relevance to the day to day practice of medicine, attending drug company sponsored seminars, which are basically sophisticated commercial events, sleeping through teleconferences, and having a fleeting affair with cyberspace. The sad thing is that little, if any credit is given to writing a paper, teaching, quality based medical staff activities, and reading. Technophysicians often attend short courses where they learn how to do a procedure. This isn't necessarily bad if the procedure is an extension or modification of procedures that were part of the physicians basic training, but when this is not the case, when it is obviously geared to provide the physician with lucrative gimmicks.

This isn't rocket science. I will bet that all physicians will admit that their learning experience in medical school was efficient and durable. Maybe it was arduous, but necessary, and accepted as the path to take to become a physician. I don't know anyone who sloughed off during medical school, or who was comfortable with a gentleman's C. The activity was focused, with lecture material, supported by relevant reading and the laboratory experience. Significant motivators at that particular stage of development were the threat of failure, which implied not becoming a doctor, or the quest for higher grades, which opened up the better internships and residencies. Is striving to practice high quality medicine less important? It seems so.

Graduation bestows the title of doctor but seems to relieve technophysicias of the effort of study. Is this right? Residencies and fellowships are usually experiential, with less reading and fewer lectures, and often designed to hone the skills of technophysicians. Is it inappropriate to expect technophysicians to periodically return to the classroom to stay current? I'll let the reader by the judge.

Two examples come to mind: The clinical pathological conference and the mortality-morbidity conference represent two tried and tested formats providing an educational experience for medical students, house officers, and practicing physicians. A model CPC continues to be faithfully published in *The New England Journal of Medicine.* The reader or attendee is treated to an unknown medical problem, which is solved by an expert clinician. A diagnosis is made after analyzing all of the data, reviewing pertinent literature, and weaving all of this into personal experience. This is confirmed or rejected by the pathological exam, the final arbiter. This format is easily usable at the community hospital level. But that doesn't happen.

The mortality-morbidity format deals honestly with unexpected outcomes or complications, analyzing what went wrong, and what to do with a similar case next time. One might presuppose that technophysicians would continue with this format in their local hospitals. Not so. Again, no interest. No time. No need.

In the first instance, the CPC requires reading, studying, and risk taking. These appear to lost arts. In the second, there is the assumption of honesty; that physicians who have less than desirable outcomes or complications would be interested in presenting their experience and look for help from their colleagues. Not so. Malpractice exposure is the usual disclaimer. This cowardly attitude has doomed the M & M experience. A few brave souls make the effort to attend the weekly CPC or M&M events at the local medical school. Most of these conferences are woefully under attended by outside physicians. The audience is primarily composed of medical students and house officers, which is quite appropriate, yet there is room and a standing invitation for outside physicians to get involved. Taking a risk, offering an opinion, sharing experience, being on the spot, are not activities sought after by practicing physicians. Perhaps these experiences were hated during the training process. Perhaps many physicians take criticism personally. Perhaps physicians are afraid of having their weaknesses exposed, even though this is a pathway to strength. For whatever reason, physicians are not involved and the opportunity for a great learning experience is lost.

Most of the educational activity that takes place in the lives of practicing physicians has more to do with learning how to master new gimmicks, which define the nature of technophyicians, or simply attending some nonsense course that fulfills the statutory obligation for CME credits. Basic science advances, which grow from the body of established knowledge, are left to the teachers and researchers. Obviously, to understand and follow scientific inquiry, there is a need to constantly review and relearn known truths, as well as the advances, which are the substrate from which scientific advancement arises.

Digestive Disease Week sponsored by the American Gastroenterology Association is a favorite of mine. This has been bifurcated into two conferences, one for the physician scientists and one for the practicing clinicians. This is not necessarily a bad idea. The slogan is "from bench to bedside", presenting relevant scientific discoveries which promise clinical usefulness. As previously discussed, the gulf that separates science from technomedicine, has become a major impediment to quality and meaningful health care.

One of the most popular attractions at DDW is the display of new technology, a carnival of sorts, just outside the main lecture rooms. This is where decisions are made to lobby hospitals to procure expensive technology to satisfy the technophysicians. This is where the technophysician plans his assault on the local hospital administration to convince these persons about the usefulness and profitability of a new and expensive device. If these new gadgets had scientific validity, that would be one thing. But, in part because of a loophole in the FDA approval process, many of these devices have not been carefully studied. So, technophysicians are willing to try out relatively untested technology on unsuspecting patients.

Turf protection, power, and economics all drive technophysicians to subordinate a meaningful educational experience to avarice, an attitude that has not only become part of the medical school curricula, but is also woven into the fabric of private practice. Many patients in community hospitals unknowingly become part of the training process for new and difficult procedures, often untested as to efficacy and clinical outcomes, placing these unsuspecting patients in harm's way, at the same time contributing mightily to health care expenditures. The most unsettling part of this is that technophysicians often learn these new techniques from sales persons.

Meaningful continuing medical education is more than entertainment; it is a personal odyssey that leads to excellence. It is an integral part of the service aspect of practicing medicine. A well educated physician is better able to explain the reasons for a particular diagnostic or therapeutic intervention, the cause of disease or ill health, the reasons for "pulling the plug", and the understanding of symptoms. Patients are made better partners in the health care drama. Patients are provided with the opportunity to become advocates for meaningful health care endeavors.

At one time during my involvement with the department of gastroenterology at UC Davis, I attempted to broker a relationship between the university and our local hospital. We had a number of excellent gastroenterologists and my thought was that a town-gown synthesis would be worthwhile. UC Davis Medical Center is located in the old Sacramento County Hospital, and, as such, has a clientele that reflects many of the inner city have-nots. It is a truism that the patients seen in large county or charity hospitals present a different spectrum of health care issues, often consequences of lifestyle and their pitiful socioeconomic circumstance. The physician-in-training is often over-trained in this arena and needs exposure to "middle class medicine." The disease mix seen at our community hospital was a repository of challenging cases, which promised an additional education experience for these new gastroenterologists. The department of gastroenterology and the medical school in general signed off on the proposal. Our community hospital signed off. The nurses in our department were excited about the prospect of being involved in a learning experience for budding gastroenterologists. The deal fell through, however. Why? My colleagues at the community hospital were not inclined to help train new gastroenterologists who were potential competitors. The educational benefits to all were eclipsed by self-interest. This very human character defect became the ignominious deal breaker.

The teaching of medical students and house officers has been one of the most rewarding educational experiences that I have ever had. The interaction demands honesty and a focus, which engages the instructor in the process of continual study. The rewards are incalculable; an interaction and exchange of information with students that hones the instructor's fund of knowledge and insures a higher quality for his own practice. I spent nearly 20 years on the voluntary faculty at UC Davis, rising from a clinical instructor to a full clinical professor. These titles are mostly honorary but they do attest to a certain commitment, which I am proud to have had. My mismanagement of Hank motivated me to get involved. My own experiences included various exposures to the medical educational process: lecturing medical students, participating in clinical pathological conferences, participating in the teaching of endoscopy to GI fellows, organizing and teaching third year surgical residents the basics of endoscopy, and running a clinical gastroenterology clinic for third year medical residents. These were challenging tasks but what I learned was far more than I passed on. A private physician, often called an attending, gives of his time to participate in the education of young doctors. It is an honor, but at the same time, it requires preparation, time away from one's practice, and a willingness to be part of the drama of learning, with the exhilaration and frustrations, the highs and lows, the successes and failures. My own belief is that physicians who give their time to participate in this process tend to be the better doctors.

The end of my involvement with teaching at the medical school was a shock. Over the years I had been grateful for the enthusiastic appraisals of my work by students and fellow faculty. I had been chosen to be a member of the joint voluntary faculty and paid faculty committee to plan and further medical education. I had even been invited to consider becoming a full time faculty person. These were honors that I greatly appreciated.

It came out of the blue. The timing was unbelievable. There had been some discussion about reorganizing the primary care clinic, which included mine. The focus of my clinic had been to offer residents a different view of problem solving, an invitation to use the time honored patient's history and bedside evaluation to understand the mechanism of disease, and choose a therapeutic path that did not automatically lead to an invasive study. I tried to share some of my experience with the art of medicine, the nature of empathy, the importance of communication, and the ability to discern those cases that demanded urgent and aggressive care versus cases which could be handled more simply. Most of the cases I discussed with the residents didn't need endoscopy or any other intrusive study. However, there were other considerations being discussed by those in charge of the curricula. Although I have no facts to support it, I believe there was concern that my clinic was not a moneymaker. When I opened the envelope the words that hurt the most were "*services not needed.*" Here I was a voluntary teacher, being essentially fired.

I had been fired once previously. When I was 14 years old I got a job cutting the church lawn. The grounds manager, Lars Olson, who was a total asshole, or at least that's my recollection, constantly got into my face about this and that. So, behaving like a typical adolescent, I told him to go fuck himself. In a second, I was gone. In retrospect, I have come to understand what happened and my part in it. But, getting a "pink-slip" from a place where I felt honored to give of my time, continues to be difficult to understand.

This experience was an up close and personal look at the economics of health care. I learned that generating invasive tests trumped the educational process. There is certainly an educational experience in learning how to do a procedure, but it is so closely connected to the ultimate monitory rewards that the experience is adulterated. There are certainly better teachers than me, but few that feel more strongly about the educational experience. There was never any personal communication from the higher-ups. I stood in a void, surrounded by uncertainty, disappointment, and betrayal. This was the closest I had ever come to the political machinations of the full time faculty. The advantage of being an outside voluntary faculty person provided a certain freedom from the tedious constraints of the political infighting so characteristic of academe. At the same time, I had little, if any influence, watching the educational process drift further in the direction of technophysicians.

The "real politic" of quality in the medical school has had great influence in the community hospital experience. The vast majority of health care decision-making in our country occurs in smaller community hospitals, which stretch throughout suburbia, across the nation, standing as beacons for the extension of high tech medicine to every corner of the nation. These community hospitals are now infiltrated by technophysicians who reflect the insouciant attitudes that characterize their faculty. Cynicism and a plethoric revenue stream have spread from the medical school to the periphery, subordinating the healing experience to the financial rewards and the glitter of high tech medicine. It's bad enough that technophysicians have less time or inclination to read, given their commitment to enhance their incomes by working harder, but now many authors whose review articles appear in prestigious journals, like the New England Journal of Medicine, actually have significant financial relationships and ties with the health care industry, whose job it is to promote drugs and medical devices. This conflict of interest is not readily apparent to the unsuspecting medical conference attendee when the disclosure effort if feeble.

Add to this the fact that big pharma underwrites much of the CME effort and you see what I'm talking about. The hegemony that academia has traditionally had over CME has been attenuated or totally eclipsed by big pharma, which now underwrites much of the activity, certainly a break for physicians, but injecting subtle bias into the process. Lectures are sprinkled with subliminal references to the advisability of using their products. This is where the fruit from the forbidden tree becomes irresistible to many technophysicians who often feel that they are entitled to these perks since their incomes have decreased. Medical schools and professional societies disingenuously complain that they would be unable to finance CME activities without support from industry. Industry bias seems much worse to me than fewer quality conferences. Medical schools seem more interested in engaging in the orgy of high tech medicine, because of the significant financial rewards from doing procedures and the profits from developing a new drug, treatment, or device. It is unadulterated greed, invading and destroying the notion of quality.

We technophysicians have acquiesced and bought in to these dangerous new trends since the number of perks, the number of free seminars, and hefty stipends for our own time as speakers, is alluring and irresistible. According to Public Citizen, a watchdog organization in Washington, DC, the yearly revenues for commercial CME suppliers are more than 600 million dollars, and it is growing. Approximately three-quarters of the income of these commercial companies are derived from pharmaceutical companies. Although doctors still spend their some of their own money on CME to help study for board examinations, the commercial suppliers offer much of the educational material free, a sure invitation for bias, which lasts a life-time So, although participating in meaningful continuing education is not high on the technophysician's wish list, when these doctors make an attempt at meaningful CME, they are bombarded by the commercially directed information or physician-teachers with huge conflicts of interest that inculcate a profit motif for quality.

There is no inclination by the industrial-health behemoth to change this sorry state of affairs. But, this needs to be changed. Physicians should voluntarily involve themselves with meaningful continuing education, but they don't. Medical schools should allow and encourage practicing physicians to take time off from their busy practices in order to return to these citadels of learning, but they don't. I believe efforts should be made by medical schools to integrate interested physicians with interns and residents as part of the medical school's commitment to education. If developed properly, this one or two month respite from the rigors of private practice would be traded in for a robust educational experience, using the format that all physicians remember from training days. The practicing physician would be given the opportunity to keep abreast of new information, and at the same time transfer wisdom to developing physicians. I suspect that the costs would inevitably be born by the practicing physician, but it seems like a worthwhile investment. Diplomas or attestations could be awarded to these committed practicing physicians that might serve as a reference source for patients looking for good doctors. Will this ever happen? If it were demanded by all of us, by the citizenry, it would. I will discuss this in the final chapter.

Chapter 10
Professionalism: An Endangered Species

The macho feel of the operating room is not unlike that of a baseball diamond, a football field, or a basketball court. Scrub nurses and circulating nurses are often female, but they adjust to the male atmosphere, if for no other reason than to keep their jobs. The lights are bright; the whole place is awash in antisepsis punctuated by sterile green drapes. The surgeon, as well as the rest of the cast, wears the familiar gowns with gloves, masks, hats and paper booties slipped over shoes. A certain freedom reigns when the patient is asleep. The surgical team can then be real, or silly, or vulgar. Some of the best and worst of human nature is on display in the highly charged operating room. The focus is usually on the surgical incision and what lies below, but the laparoscopic technique creates some displacement of the in situ experience. Everything is seen on a video screen, a surrealistic representation of tissue and plasma, an other world dimension. The task of the surgeon is to correctly identify the various structures, all to be done without the benefit of actually feeling these structures, heretofore an important tactile requirement for the general surgeon.

In the background there is the music of the breathing apparatus that sustains the patient, the bright lights on the computerized console guiding the anesthesiologist (much as visual screens do for air-traffic controllers), and the give-and-take banter between the surgeon, his assistant and the various nurses. A large tray contains the vast assortment of instruments used by the physicians, and woe be it to the unlucky person who contaminates these! Sterile technique is so important. We have Pasteur and Koch to thank for this. How one washes or scrubs, how the gowns and gloves are put on, how a person moves about avoiding the sterile areas are all parts of the symphony of decontamination.

This was a busy day for Jason Moody. Dr. Moody was a general surgeon who had found himself marginalized over the years because there were other surgeons who were brighter, more skilled, and more affable. Jason had been around for quite awhile, often assisting since that was one way to pay the bills, but never really very busy. There are usually far more surgeons in any given area than surgeries needed. So, this second tier, where Jason resided, satisfies itself with leftovers, simple procedures that the first tier disdains, and assisting.

Jason's day was busy because he had family matters, a sick relative, a neurasthenic wife, unruly children, and more office patients than he had expected. Today's surgery had been scheduled for one PM, but Jason was a good thirty minutes late. Nothing so disrupts a busy operating room schedule than a late surgeon, especially one who belongs to the second tier. The nurses mumble amongst themselves, the first tier surgeons rant and rave, and the anesthesiologist is thrown out of rhythm. No one is happy, especially the patient, who is beside himself in the holding area, surrounded by nervous relatives, all wondering why.

Jason flew through the operating area door and quickly headed for the male dressing room. He left a trail of discontent in his wake. At the same time the orderlies moved his patient into the designated operating room, ushering the family to the proper waiting area, which sent the signal that the other players were to move into place. This was all done rather quickly in part to placate the other surgeons who were forced to wait in line.

Jason sheepishly entered the designated operating room, made a perfunctory attempt to apologize, and was assisted in drying his recently scrubbed hands. The general atmosphere was tense. The anesthesiologist wisely started pre anesthesia sedation to spare the poor patient from the room's toxicity. This was to be a laparoscopic cholecystectomy, a surgical technique to remove the gallbladder.

For many years a formal cholecystectomy meant several days in the hospital and several weeks of convalescence. No more. Now patients can be operated upon and discharged within twenty-four hours. These happy souls are often back at work in several days. Five small abdominal scars have come to replace the traditional long, right upper-quadrant scar. The modern surgery is less costly, probably a little safer, less painful, and the outcomes of the laparoscopic method are usually better than those of the conventional operation, depending upon how skilled the surgeon is. The down side of all of this has been that while new surgeons have a great deal of experience mastering the laparoscopic methodology, they have much less with the traditional open cholecystectomy. It is mandatory to be skilled at converting to the open method if there are complications, or likely to be complications. Unfortunately, not all of these new technophysician surgeons are capable of seamlessly converting to the open method. Such was the case with Dr. Moody, which must have always been in the back of his mind. Once in the OR the task is to pass a laparoscope through the abdominal wall after the abdominal cavity was filled with gas. Surgeons use noninflammable carbon dioxide, which allows the use of a cautery to remove gall bladders, tumors or repair hernias. With the scope in place, the liver can be easily studied, a dispassionate consideration of what Galen thought was where pneuma (air), the life breath of the cosmos, was modified and became the nutritive soul that supported the vegetative function of growth and nutrition. Galen believed that this was done by way of the veins that originated in the liver. I'm not sure if Galen appreciated the fact that bile was synthesized in the liver, and stored in the gallbladder, and if the gallbladder developed stones, any number of problems could develop. It's probably just as well that Galen didn't have access to laparoscopy.

Shortly after the patient was properly anesthetized, Moody made the requisite five incisions, put a trochar into the abdominal cavity and began to insufflate with gas. When he reached for the laparoscope it was not in the usual location on the instrument tray where he was accustomed to having it; a minor error, but Jason was in no shape for even a minor error. Jason inadvertently contaminated the other instruments on the tray. His level of internal discomfort must have soared mightily, his self-control melted away, all of his transitory life's problems crashed upon him, and he acted out. He suddenly grabbed a bloody towel and threw it across the patient at the scrub nurse hitting him in the face and knocking his glasses off. Jason regained control of himself, the scrub nurse excused himself, and the procedure was successfully completed. But Jason's troubles were just starting.

Nearly at the end of my three-year term as chief-of-staff, my hope was that nothing more would happen until January 1 when I passed the gauntlet. But I was wrong. This case was a little different. The year was 1993. All of us understood that blood was a potential lethal weapon given the number of blood borne viruses, which were wrecking havoc. This was an assault and there was the threat of a criminal action, a suit, and

God-knows what else. Here was an opportunity for the medical staff to appropriately discipline a member who had crossed the line.

Moody was initially suspended for 7 days by the department of surgery. The point was to do something, but not enough to have him reported to the National Physician's Data Bank, which would leave an indelible mark against his name for perpetuity. Anything over 7 days would have triggered consequences for Dr. Moody, which were significant. A physician's good name was more important to his colleagues than protecting the public. The Board of Trustees was hopping mad and needed more than this. They needed information. The board of trustees at any hospital is the final authority over the practice of medicine. The board needed to know how this happened and what meaningful punishment was the medical staff going to mete out. That body was all too aware that this case could turn into a public relations nightmare should the aggrieved nurse speak out. They were aware that the district attorney could get involved as there was reason to consider criminal assault and other less savory legal injunctions. None of this girded the loins of the medical executive committee, which took exception to the notion that the hospital board of trust was meddling in their affairs. The MEC entrenched itself, defied outside advice, and made a feeble attempt at conducting an impartial investigation.

Other nurses who were in the OR with Moody were asked to "testify." They were frightened, confused, but tearfully recounted the events of that day. Moody also gave his side of the story and rested his case on the declaration that he didn't mean to do it. The MEC weighed the potential cost to Dr. Moody with respect to his reputation and future professional success vs. the nature of the event—Was it intentional? Did it cause any harm? Had Moody ever done something like this before? Was his apology to the nurse sufficient? Did he need psychological counseling? The MEC essentially sided with Moody. It would confine itself to the 7- day suspension. The MEC was in no mood to cave in to the implicit wishes of the board of trustees. The MEC rallied around one of its own, protected him, insulated him, and lost an opportunity to gain the professional high ground. So, Moody "served" his 7-day suspension, returned to work as if nothing happened, and, unknown to the general public represented a potential threat to their future welfare. If a surgeon is so out of control that he flings a contaminated towel across the room, then it doesn't take much imagination to wonder what else he might do that may be a threat to a patient. The nurse victim went silent, never to utter a word about the debacle. The case was closed.

This is not an isolated incident. It happens all of the time within the confines of medical staffs across the country. The medical staffs perceive themselves under siege by attorneys, the government, the hospital, and anyone else who is interested in regulating medicine. Never mind that physicians are the only ones who can write orders and thus are ultimately responsible for the health of us all. Never mind that physician behavior contributes mightily to the escalating costs of health care. Never mind that indifference to the underpinnings of professionalism is eroding away the very nature of quality health care in America. We physicians are simply asking to be regulated, and that is frightening since the regulators promise more mischief than is already present.

Let me tell you another story, one that peels away the veneer of propriety, which physician inherit when they become a doctor, This event occurred about the time of Jason's troubles. As the chief-or-staff, I was asked to convene the physicians health committee. This committee deals with issues such as alcoholism and drug abuse amongst physicians, unethical behavior and anger management to name a few. A lady anesthesiologist was asked to appear to explain an unusual circumstance. She was distraught, angry, and embarrassed. She had been on the staff for many years, was near retiring and had an excellent reputation. As a female she was made to endure the macho atmosphere in the operating for many years, never complaining, just doing her job like a professional. She probably had more than one instance where she could legitimately raise the issue of sexual harassment in the workplace, but knowing her, she appreciated being part of the surgical team and being part or the drama of surgery, Some of the nurses brought this issue to our attention. They recalled her asking to be excused to go the restroom. Ordinarily, this would be easy enough, another anesthesiologist would spell her and the surgeon, of course, would make sure this happened. Not on this particular day. The surgeon relied on her expertise, felt that he needed her to be present, and told her not to go. She could have made a scene, demanding to go, but she didn't because her commitment to professionalism eclipsed nature. The nurses, however, were disturbed that a pool of urine suddenly appeared around the head of the table, where the anesthesiologist worked, and suddenly engulfed their feet. So, it appeared that she simply urinated on the floor. This was an extraordinarily unusual situation, one that I had never heard of before, and begged a number of questions that were put to her. She responded, somewhat tearfully, that she didn't want to leave because of the surgeons admonition and because of her incontinence she had no other choice. The spotlight seemed to be on the wrong person. In fact it was and our next meeting of the physicians health committee dealt with the insensitive physician, who happened to be a technophysician, and a prototypically self-centered bastard. Professionalism only works when all the physicians on a team are on the same page. Behavior like this is born from the insensitivity that we are bathed in during the process of becoming a doctor. It is simply a gauge of the degree of indifference so often a part of a technophysician's make-up, an assault of professionalism. Professionalism rests on the bedrock of self-governance and self-regulation. If these elements are not in place the industry is a house of cards. Professionalism is a sure casualty of technophysicians gone wild.

There has been some interest in doing away with this staff model of self governance. This would inevitably entrench laypersons, health care engineers into the process, which would include peer review, amongst other physician responsibilities. It would be a catastrophic mistake; instilling task oriented laypersons with the mandate to regulate an honorable vocation. This would be the ultimate in government control, decimating a self-governance system, albeit there is certainly room for improvement by doctors. Is the best we can do? I think not.

The excesses of the last half of the 20th century have made professionalism an endangered species. Physicians have misused their self-governance and self-regulation, much as they did with Dr. Moody and the lady anesthesiologist, seduced by pride, control, and rewards, and are now responsible for the free fall into the health care crisis. But, there's more to professionalism than this.

Free care is at the core of any definition of professionalism. When physicians voluntarily give of their free time it is an example of service in living color. Dr. George Lundberg, the highly respected and former editor of the *Journal of the American Medical Association,* estimates that nearly one third of the physician population intentionally offer no free care at all, declining to attend free clinics or hospitals. My experience is that the number is higher. It is the exception, rather than the rule, that doctors give of their free time. The reasons for this are multiple: discounted fee for service suffices, the government already gets its share of free care with MediCare and MediCaid; charity patients are more likely to sue; managed care leaves little time for free care. The list goes on and on.

Several years ago, when I was living in Sacramento, I had the privilege of participating in the development of a free clinic. All comers were accepted in this under served neighborhood. There was no requirement for insurance attestation or green cards. There were certainly some MediCaid patients who took unfair advantage of our open door policy, and inevitably some illegal aliens queued up as well. The focus was providing basic health care to those individuals who were not insured. Many of these folks had jobs but made too much money for MediCaid and too little for health insurance premiums.

I had never participated in a free clinic outside of my training experience at Los Angeles County General Hospital. Los Angeles County General Hospital was one of a number of large teaching, charity hospitals that characterized the landscape during the years before and after World War II. This was an era when philanthropy was king, when poor patients were always assured of a hospital bed, albeit this was often a ward bed with few if any amenities.

Our free clinic represented the first time I personally decided to give free care to under served patients. It was an active choice, not because of the prevailing dogma, not because some insurance company or the government decided to discount my fee for service, not done because it was part of my training program, and not done occasionally, but on a continuing basis. There were accolades by nurses, paramedical personnel, the patients, and some friends, but the greatest thrill of all was in just doing it because I had decided to do it. Until that time I had never made a conscious decision to participate in the care of poor people. I had certainly cared for poor people during training, but it was not my decision. I had indirectly done it with discounted fee for service, but it was not my decision. I was involved with this project for several years before I moved to Hawaii.

The clinic was Thursday evening. During the winter months the cold weather, the fog, rain, and the fatigue after a day's work, often gave me pause to consider my decision. But, the feeling after the clinic was over, after seeing so many smiling and grateful faces, was more than worth the effort. I really felt like a doctor. There was some initial apprehension about the need to put away my technophysician instincts and focus on general medicine, using common sense, ministering to these patients without resorting to high technology. These concerns took care of themselves.

Our facility was in a small trailer in a low-income area. Our patients were Russian, Polish, Mexican, and Southeast Asian immigrants who lived in the area. It took a while before we earned their confidence, but with patience, it happened. Our clinic was primarily geared to deal with patients with episodic medical problems who did not have access to health care. To follow up with these patients, we established relationships with area specialists who gave their time.

The question asked by my colleagues was why a free clinic? Don't physicians already provide a great deal of free care? The answer to this question was, of course, "Yes." Discounted fee-for-service and prepaid insurance plans have led to much uncompensated physician service. Virtually all payers or insurance companies, reduce the amount a physician actually receives to a fraction of what he charges. If one were inclined to keep score, there is no question but that physicians contribute a large sum of money to charity. State and federal agencies have somewhat arbitrarily whittled away at the physician's fee during the past generation and have essentially balanced their books on the physician's back. President Obama has suggested cutting back on Medicare as part of his proposed reorganization of health care dollars. This would include physician salaries, which are often the focus for governmental or industry efforts to reduce health care expenditures. In actuality, physicians have no room to complain given the fact that they are the ones who have driven up the cost of health care. Yet, physicians have accepted this—albeit, often unwillingly—as a necessary price to pay for these escalating costs. So why do we need a free clinic?

For those who give of their time and talents there is a validation of that initial commitment to a career in medicine. For just a moment, the rust that may have encased that golden kernel of altruism is swept away, the physician is rejuvenated, and health care in America is well served.

I recall the beaming faces of patients who were totally amazed that there was professional care for them. I didn't have to speak the language to understand that they were very grateful: the new mother who didn't know how to nurse her infant; the gardener who didn't understand how important it was to drink water; the teenager who didn't know how to prevent a pregnancy; the diabetic who was amazed how important it was to control her blood sugar; the frightened child whose earache improved with medicine ; and most especially, the children of immigrants, who had become bilingual and served with pride as translators for their parents. Their gifts to me were much more than mine to them, especially given the fact that I was a technophysician, a technophysician whose professional existence was defined by a gimmick, a diagnostic or therapeutic tool, such as a gastroscope, which if used inappropriately becomes a gimmick.

Another defining characteristic of professionalism is the willingness to teach, to give time to the education of medical students or young physicians, giving back some of what had been given to us. These are not requirements for practicing physicians, rather a commitment to serve both physicians-in-training, as well as charity patients. Had it not been for those attending, voluntary physicians, willing to participate in our education, the outcome would have been less certain. The admitting schedule at Los Angeles County General Hospital for interns and residents was overwhelming. After 36 hours of admitting and caring for the sick and destitute of Los Angeles, we house officers were totally fatigued, ill mannered, unshaven, and malodorous. In the midst of finishing our shifts, the morning after, we were to present the patients, their symptoms, physical findings, and lab work to faculty, many of whom were called "attending", usually private practitioners who volunteered their time to teach us. I usually resented having to stop and "entertain" these doctors, who were carefully dressed in expensive suits, well manicured and coiffed, bathed in fine soaps and colognes. We were so disheveled, tired, and stinky, that it must have been an abominable chore for these men and women. But they stayed the course. This is where we learned much of the magic and mystery of healing, this is where we were allowed to see the end of the tunnel. It was their teaching, their commitment to voluntarily help us sort all of this mess that I have ultimately come to appreciate. They were there for us, never complaining, never short changing us, providing us with shoulders to stand on as we became more proficient doctors.

Greed has trumped professionalism. Ironically, the arrival of MediCare and MediCaid in 1965 paved the way for the escalation of physician greed. The federal government began to subsidize the development of technophysicians. Clinical services replaced research and teaching as the medical school's primary mission when these governmental programs began paying faculty a generous fee-for-service for taking care of MediCare and MediCaid patients. Greed sprouted in medical schools, a contagion that spread to residents learning how the play the keyboard of high technology. Charity hospitals and charity medicine took it in the shorts with the migration of these patients to community hospitals. Physicians could feel justified since the federal government was leading the band, subsidizing the development of technophysicians, at the same time paying for their services in community hospitals. Greed trumped professionalism, greed dressed up as medical advancement; greed camouflaged as providing the latest and most advanced care, and we patients bought it.

At the heart of professionalism is honesty. I have already spoken of physician attitudes toward peer review. Honesty is also eclipsed by self-interest, financial gain, and greed. Honesty presupposes that physicians own up to their complications, allowing their experience to serve as a template for learning, for not making the same mistake again, and helping others avoid the same pitfall. The major hue and cry from physicians is that it would expose them to malpractice. This is not only cowardly, but also unlikely. Physicians are imbued with pomposity. We come to believe that we are nearly infallible, above criticism, and totally competent. To bare one's soul would be tantamount to admitting that human frailty was part of our makeup. As a consequence, much of what goes wrong, many of the mistakes, are simply swept under the rug. Physicians are expert at hiding their mistakes. When they can't, it occasionally results in a malpractice event, but even that event often occurs out of the view of the medical staff. Instead of the medical staff being given a chance to take advantage of an opportunity to improve, there is simply hushed conversation in the doctor's dining room about some poor bastard's plight when malpractice is an issue. This was certainly my experience with Hank. Many of these cases never see the light of day in the peer review process because of the burial approach. All of us gather around to protect a colleague and indirectly cosign the dishonesty.

It is variously estimated that between 44,000 and 98,000 hospital deaths occur each year due to medical mistakes and mishaps. Much of this is systemic, i.e. poor physician handwriting, poor communication, a lack of leadership, technical failures, and health care delivery processes that are vague, outdated, or simply not there. Still, it is the physician who writes the order, who is ultimately responsible, and who must be accountable. Clear cut physician errors occur: the wrong dose of a drug, or the wrong drug, a failure to closely follow a critical patient's course, a misinterpretation of data, a failure to obtain appropriate consultation, and performing procedures in a sloppy fashion.

Yet, during my three years as a chief of staff only a handful of these cases reached the MEC or my office. So, if medical mistakes account for such a sizeable toll of hospital deaths, or injury, there must be a lot of burying going on. And, there is. Many of the malpractice events would go away with honesty. Many family members sue because they are angry that there is no communication, that a cover up is suspected, that an honest effort is not being made by the medical staff and the involved physician to improve. The need to protect one's self, to hide deficiencies, to avoid confrontation, all account for this stealth on the part of the physicians. The underlying issue is greed. Physicians, especially technophysicians, always want to put on their best face in order to maintain their reputation and continue to get referrals. This is so imbedded within the matrix of the medical staff's behavior that we physicians have stood aside and allowed the winds of change to indiscriminately drive up health care expenditures.

Finally, there is the issue of specialty backup of emergency room coverage. In other words, the task was to divine a way for technophysicians to help out when the problem was over the head of the ER doctor. As a chief-of-staff, one of the most distasteful issues for me was insuring that this backup coverage was intact. A new breed of doctor now assumes primary coverage, physicians who are properly trained to deal with the ER patient, where the spectrum of illness ranges from shock to anxiety. These are highly trained physicians, board certified, who have been trained to insure that the initial response for sick patients is competent. They are on site for 24/7, providing hospitals with continuous professional service. But, they need backup coverage. If it is head injury, a trauma case, a bowel obstruction, a woman with prolonged labor, or a gastrointestinal bleed, the ER physician needs help, and the expectation is that help is available. This "expectation" was a big issue, as physicians are much less inclined to lend a hand. They understandingly resent getting out of bed, working through the night, having to cancel the next day, and not getting paid. But the root cause of this reflects back on the dysfunctional point of service, where technophysicians have distained healing medicine.

Years ago I took care of the father of a lawyer friend of mine. He was hospitalized with advanced pancreatic carcinoma. He struggled during the final month of his life with abdominal pain and progressive jaundice. It was concluded that his disease was so far advanced that surgery was out of the question. Chemotherapy, which has always been limited in this disease, was declined by the patient. During his last hospitalization he had a significant gastrointestinal bleed. His will to survive was formidable; he fought every step of the way. His son and I explained that it was a futile situation, in spite of the fact that hope was always appropriate. He had trouble with this. When the end came he was surrounded by his son, myself, two nurses, a case manager, and a nun. We all held hands and recited the 23rd psalm. He gave up the fight, he released, and quietly passed away. There were tears in all or our eyes, but the dignity of death was given its due and put a healing touch on the inevitable. But, with technophysicians, the focus is changed, the expectations are different, and so, resentments, indifference, and hostility have their way, and once again, professionalism is decimated.

Professionalism is one of the bedrocks from which healing springs. Sadly, it is becoming a lost art, unable to compete with technophysicians, where there is no time or inclination to become involved. If power, control and greed are the rings on the merry go-round, then what value does professionalism play? There is little interest.

But how to get the technophysicians involved? Traditionally, professionalism has included covering the community hospital ER as part of giving something back to the community. With discounted fee for service, an increase in malpractice events, and government intrusion into the practice of medicine, many doctors no longer feel obliged or inclined to cover the ER. Technophysicians complain that their services are uncompensated, that there is increased exposure to malpractice, and that it's basically the hospital's responsibility. The medical staff bylaws assume that all specialties are covered, so if a technophysician refuses to take call, this becomes an issue.

If a child contracts epiglottitis, a medical emergency where the epiglottis in inflamed by the bacterium Hemophilus influenzae, and where the air way becomes obstructed and breathing becomes impossible because of this enlarged, edematous, and inflamed epiglottis, antibiotics are helpful but they don't work fast enough. The standard treatment is to have an ENT doctor perform an emergency tracheotomy, a life-saving procedure, and well within an ENT's privileged list of procedures. Getting ENT doctors to provide backup specialty call was nearly impossible. Granted, epiglottitis is rare, but it does occur, and this, as well as other ENT emergencies occur, frequently or not. Our ENT physicians argued that they really didn't need to on the active medical staff since most of their work was in their offices; thus the medical bylaws verbiage regarding coverage was moot, and besides they were now busy with outpatient plastic surgery and they didn't feel competent to do an emergency tracheotomy. This seemed not only disingenuous, but a cop-out.

Technophysicians are expert at dodging the issue and the organized medical staff is often impotent at enforcing back-up call. At my hospital the way out of this problem was to throw money at it. By paying highly trained technophysicians a stipend for on call duty, the hospital solved the problem. Note that the hospital's solution did not speak to professionalism. Our hospital administration's decision was pragmatic, made for financial and legal reasons, which put a price tag on altruism and service. Remuneration trumped professionalism, where community service was a higher calling. Paying back-up technophysicians solved the problem, it worked, and coverage was complete. But it was done in the absence of professionalism, a certain casualty for genuine health care.

It is abundantly true that the remuneration for dealing with an after hours emergency is woefully insufficient. I do believe that coming in during the middle of the night to treat a patient should be rewarded monetarily, at least much better than presently exists. I believe that there is money to do this, but it supposes that unnecessary procedures are eliminated. I will have more to say about that.

Honesty, quality, integrity, and service are ballast for professionalism. Sadly, these qualities are slowly eroding, paving the way for impersonal, conveyer belt medicine, which is exactly what we patients will get in spades if single payer or national health scheme becomes operative or is we don't demand more from our physicians. We must hold physicians to the highest standards if they want our business. Time is of the essence. If physicians are not persuaded to make significant and fundamental changes in their practice of medicine, then all of us will be left with a government solution guaranteed to infuse mediocrity. Mediocrity would affect all layers of the health care experience. Honestly motivated clinicians would be drowned by paper work ostensibly justifying their medical decisions. Some of this goes on today with payers declining services felt to be too expensive, where decisions are made on financial grounds rather than quality based terms. This would be magnified if he government were the sole payer, where cost control would eclipse quality, where health care engineers would be calling the shots. This is a people problem.

To recapitulate, these two areas, namely continuing medical education and professionalism, have been decimated by technophysicians and will become an endangered species with governmental sponsored single payer or managed care. I presently live and practice in Hawaii. This has been an up close and personal vantage point from which to view single payer medicine. Hawaii has mandated that employers pay health insurance for their employees, and the methodology has been to select HMSA, a derivation of Blue Cross/ Blue Shield, to more or less be the state's single payer. I can tell you that this had a major adverse impact on physician morale, motivation, and incentive. This is a very heavy handed state, that has its fingers in nearly every aspect of health care, and the result is a shortage of physicians, difficulty in recruiting physicians, and physicians leaving for the mainland. To be fair, the high cost of living and tort reform issues play a role, but the draconian efforts of HMSA is the major issue. The real culprit is the high cost of technophysicians with their rising health care expenditures. Hawaii offers a glimpse into the future. This is a path that the federal government has attempted to define by passing ObamaCare. By expanding MediCaid and providing subsidies for the purchase of insurance, by mandating this purchase by those not covered, the government will take a big step in regulating the industry. However, the labyrinthine governmental bureaucracy, which is laden with inertia has done little to breathe life into the availability of physicians in Hawaii. Patients do have coverage, but with fewer and fewer doctors, and many doctors opting out of the HMSA covenant, those patients are left holding their insurance cards. Add to that the scandalously low stipends for physicians, and you have a situation where patients have access, but physician availability is the issue. This portends major problems in the other 49 states when and if some form of national health becomes a reality.

The story of Nigel Southworth, MD puts in living color the catastrophe wrought when the neglected stepchildren are in play at once. The next chapter throws back cover on cowardly behavior and the medical staff's impotence mixed together in an unhealthy brew.

Chapter 11 The Triumph of Cowardice Dysfunction Has Its Way

On an asshole scale of 10, Nigel Southworth was at least a 9. He gets two points for being a neurosurgeon and he earned the other 7. Born and raised in the UK, he arrived on our shores some 40 years ago. He was a walking/talking history lesson. As a living, breathing example of hauteur, class, race, and station, his demeanor helped explain the reasons why the Pilgrims came to the New World in the first place. When Nigel walked into a room, sat in on some insipid committee meeting, or rendered a medical opinion, it reminded me of the two stuffy Englishmen in the movie *Chariots Of Fire*. Solemnity and ponderousness best described him. He would have felt at home in the background of El Greco's *View Of Toledo*. And the bastard was oblique to the rays of reality. You couldn't tell him anything. He had gotten away with whatever he wanted because for years he was a cash cow for our hospital, accounting for a sizable chunk of the bottom line. He used that leverage very effectively, insisting on the latest equipment for his surgeries, being highly influential whenever a new operating room was built, and always avoiding serious peer review of his work. He could get away with murder, literally, because all of us were too intimidated to point out problems. This event occurred near the end of my stint as chief of staff, a couple of years before I moved to Hawaii.

As Nigel got older, lots of problems cropped up. Ironically, he suffered from a degenerative disease of his own cervical spine, which he decided to treat himself, making his condition worse. Since he was of the opinion that he had no peer, he found it difficult to ask and receive advice. To be fair, he had been an excellent neurosurgeon, introducing a number of surgical advances into our community. He was an overly meticulous operator, taking nearly twice as long to carry out a procedure than other neurosurgeons and demanding classical music to be played in the O.R. on top of it all. This drove his nurses crazy.

One day Nigel found himself over his head. The issue was the subject of conversation in the doctors' dining room, that "court of last resort." There were muffled whispers amongst the staff as to what was going to happen. As Chief of Staff, I had to strain my ears as my colleagues were now reluctant to gossip in front of me. Nevertheless it was clear that Nigel was circling in the vortex of scrutiny. Nigel had a third bad case. Having had two bad cases, where the patients went south, where the storm clouds of malpractice hovered, was more than most physicians could ignore. Not so with Nigel. He kept banging away, amazing us all, charming his patients, and seemingly oblivious to impending catastrophe. Insulated by his considerable ego, he found himself distanced from any suffering he had caused. Perhaps it was because his own back was betraying him, becoming a challenge, an invitation for self treatment, a measure of grandiosity. If he was worthy of his own ministrations, then his patients were entitled to no less. The fortress of his ego allowed him to reach out and manipulate others, whether patients or colleagues, but it was not a two-way street. There was no opportunity for life's vicissitudes to touch him. Like many physicians, he was possessed by the power of dissociation. He could open a skull, see a brain eaten away by tumor, a life destroyed, without the slightest of personal feeling. This, of course, is not uncommon with a busy neurosurgeon, but technophysicians have mastered the art of complete displacement or attenuation of feelings, which I believe that caring physicians possess. In the classic reductionist or mechanistic sense, this was simply a machine gone wrong.

Like many of us, he came to believe he was something special because of his technical skill. To Nigel leadership was taking a chance, trying out a new technique, being the first on the block to master a procedure, and his ego demanded that these things be done even in a relatively small community hospital. Nigel was convinced that he knew as much as full-time professors, and that he had a better chance to advance health care than those in the university. He had fantastic will power. His lengthy procedures wore out more than one scrub nurse. He simply wouldn't quit until he was satisfied. At noon the doctor's dining room was buzzing with activity. It was strewn with half-eaten sandwiches, empty milk cartons, salad-bar ingredients spilled here and there, and groups of physicians deep in conversation. The usual topics of sports, the market, politics, and managed care were displaced by the Nigel drama.

"What's the latest with Nigel?" blurted one of the anesthesiologists.

"What difference does it make, the guy can wiggle through anything," retorted a female pediatrician.

"Why pick on Nigel, he's done a lot for this goddamn hospital" shot back a general surgeon.

"The guy is out of control," responded the pediatrician

"He's the best neurosurgeon in this area. How can the hospital mess with him?" mumbled his internist friend.

"So he has a bad case or two, who doesn't?" was the response by the general surgeon.

Anesthesiologists are where you go if you really want to know what's going on in the operating room. I actually believe that they hate all surgeons, maybe because they aren't surgeons, maybe because they don't like being someone else's butt-boy. In the doctor's dining room they cluster together, unmistakable in their surgical greens, usually poring over the Wall Street Journal. They made certain that everyone within earshot learned that Nigel had a third bad case. All three of these all occurred when he was trying to carry out a new, somewhat difficult, procedure called anterior cervical spine plating.

Most physicians who are involved with patient care know how it feels when their patient has a poor outcome. If the cause is an accepted complication, the process of assuaging one's self is easier. It is far more difficult when the fault is our own. Perhaps it is a matter of case selection, or poor follow-up, of prescribing the wrong medicine, of taking risks where they needn't be taken, or not having the skill to pull it off. Our first instinct is to go over a checklist. What went wrong? Did we do something wrong? Will anybody find out? We wonder. When a peer has a problem there is certain deliciousness that it wasn't us, there is some sadness that it was him, there is a knee-jerk arousal of litigious instincts. What's the likelihood for malpractice? There is an autonomic response of self-preservation. There is an immediate rush to the bylaws. We all feel vulnerable. What happens to this poor guy could happen to any of us. There is some comfort knowing that our careers are protected by labyrinthine due process. Concern for the patient is subordinated to these other issues. That's sad, but that's the way it is. We end up caught in the web of defensive medicine, ordering expensive tests to protect our back-sides, adding immeasurably to health care costs.

Applying metallic plates over bone grafts has been around for some time, but applying them anteriorly to the cervical spine is a fairly recent development. This affords added stability to the cervical spine. Patients with cervical disk herniations, whose cervical spines are unstable, or who were thought to be at risk for poor healing of the autologous bone graft customarily applied, are candidates for this high-risk procedure.

The performance of this delicate procedure, namely, applying metal plates to the anterior cervical spine for purposes of effecting stability, is a very delicate operation requiring stereotactic imaging in order to properly place the metal screws into the vertebral facets. The spinal cord is an Achilles Heel; if it is damaged the outcome is often paraplegia. For elderly patients already suffering neurological sequelae from cervical spine instability, paraplegia would be a cruel outcome. Naturally, it was also a high paying procedure, which probably accounts for its popularity. My sense was many more of these procedures were being carried out than were indicated. A new breed of surgeon, called a back surgeon, has emerged. This highly trained individual is perhaps better suited for this procedure but this has caused consternation amongst neurosurgeons, and has led to a turf war.

The Joint Commission of Hospital Accreditation expects the medical staff to craft a single highest standard for all who are doing any particular procedure, regardless or whether they are neurosurgeons or back surgeons. Having two or three standards would allow each specialty group a degree of autonomy based on the nuances of its postdoctoral training program. However, JCAHO is quite explicit about this: it expects a single credentialing standard for each procedure throughout the hospital. Common sense supports JCAHO's position. Having two or three credentialing standards would inevitably lead to different levels of training and expertise, while the medical staff's goal is to expect the single highest standard of quality. The challenge then is to create a single standard, taking into account the different pathways that lead to this privilege, at the same time remaining independent from turf and economic issues. A very big challenge!

As I have said before, the medical staff often succumbs to the throw weight of the most established physicians. The neurosurgeons could have cared less what the JCAHO required, they were hell bent on keeping the status quo, and they were willing to impose their watered down standards for this procedure, namely the three-day cadaver course. The mechanism they chose to protect their turf was the requirement that this privilege was only available to neurosurgeons. Was that the highest standard? It depends on how one looks at it. If you believe that a training program in neurosurgery is a gift from Mt. Olympus or on a par with the Ten Commandments, then that would have carried the day. On the other hand, if one believed that the extra training and time spent by the back surgeons was a higher standard, then the gauntlet was thrown. The Joint Commission would accept the medical staff's decision, assuming it was the highest standard, a very debatable position if the neurosurgeons won the battle. And, it was a battle.

Before a single standard was chosen, the neurosurgeons jumped the gun, launching out on troubled waters, with disastrous results. The leader of this infamous group, Nigel, had an excellent reputation, having been educated in the finest neurosurgeon tradition. But it was not his skill that made him so valuable to the hospital, rather the revenue stream that he generated by virtue of his prodigious surgical activity. For years, he had made a fortune operating on the most difficult cases, with more than a modicum of success. As time moved on his judgment and skills began to fall off. But, he was the acknowledged leader of the pack and determined to lead the troops into battle. The gold standard for acquiring new skills would ordinarily be to take time away from practice, enroll for a short period at an academic health care center, and learn properly. This is rarely done. Why not? Well, to tell the truth, medical schools don't see the continuing education of physicians in the community as one of their mandates. Their time is precious, in large measure because the faculty are seeing patients and performing procedures as part of their own practices. Residents and fellows are invited to watch, and sometimes become involved, but the revenue stream is predicated on a busy and productive faculty person.

I believe there is also a hidden agenda, one that cloisters advanced procedures within the halls of academe, insuring that the revenue stream continues unabated. So, the private physician learns from one of his partners, attends a short course in the South Pacific, or has the audacity to teach himself on the job. Alternatively, a commercial medical device technician, who actually comes into the procedure room and guides the specialist through the procedure, sometimes handling the devices, teaches him. This, of course, is practicing medicine without a license, but it goes on all of the time. The audacity of the technophysician to learn this way is outlandish. The town gown relationship is often colored by greed, greed that is indigenous to both sides. Bravado and greed breeds megalomania, and there is plenty of that both within the halls of academe and within the confines of the community medical staff. The patient never knows because technophysicians are deft at giving informed consent, albeit disingenuous, while tiptoeing around the edge of this issue. The medical staff crumbles under pressure.

So, with a flick of his wrist Nigel ordered up this complicated and delicate third procedure and unless it went badly nobody would know the difference. The absolutely incredible part of this story is not so much that Nigel had the audacity to make the decision to try this technique for the third time, but that there were no adequate checks and balances within the structure of the medical staff to thwart this attempt. It was an invitation for disaster. Nigel laid claim to the legacy of authenticity handed down by organized medicine to neurosurgeons.

Nigel was now on dangerous ground. He had crossed the Rubicon and his calcified ego had no way of retreating. He was now out on a limb, there was no one to help him, as if he could ask for help, his instincts told him to push on even when the odds were not good.

According to the anesthesiologists, Nigel had one patient with a vocal cord injury and another with a perforation of the esophagus. These were well known complications, but two in such a short period of time by one surgeon usually raised a red flag. I was aware of all this because it was recently discussed at the medical executive committee. There were a number of folks who were concerned that Nigel was going to really fuck up and bring all kinds of despair on the hospital and medical staff. But, what to do with Nigel? Others had tried to warn him he was working too hard, how hard it was on his own cervical spine, how hard it was on the nurses and the anesthesiologists who were forced to spend hours watching him operate at a snail's pace. His surgical assistants didn't raise much of a fuss because they were getting paid fairly well. Nigel had been before various committees of peers during the past several years for other complications, complaints, and concerns. He simply blew them off retreating into his cocoon of superiority and subtly reminding us that he had no peers. And, no one had the guts to take him on since he was so intimidating, so well connected, so bright, and such a great contributor to the hospital's bottom line.

The Medical Executive Committee had gathered one summer night in a meeting room off the cafeteria in the basement. It was a stifling hot summer night and by the end of the meeting there were twenty hot, sweaty, grumpy doctors praying that Nigel would go away. The new hospital administrator who wanted us to do something prodded us into some sort of action. So the issue came straight to the medical executive committee, without an ad hoc investigatory committee. The medical staff bylaws

Reinvent the Heal

allowed for that option but none of the grumpy doctors were happy about it.

"Is there a motion to do something here?" I managed to say.

"We need more information." Blurted an exasperated general surgeon

"Three bad cases isn't enough?' I responded

"Hansen, this guy is too important to the hospital." was the retort by the general surgeon.

"So, are you prepared to have a go for a fourth case?" I shot back

"These are very difficult cases, anyone can have problems." Was the response of a sleepy vascular surgeon.

"Where do we draw the line? " I pleaded.

"Don't you think it's a bit extreme taking away a good man's ability to make a living?" fired back the general surgeon.

The debate went on and on. There was a decided tilt to the meeting. Most of the members gathered around Nigel to protect his good name and not interfere with his practice.

The hospital administrator had a grimace on his face. I wasn't certain if it was malcontent or gas. Beads of sweat were beginning to form on my brow. It was now nearly midnight, this was the last agenda item, we could spend another full meeting on this, but something needed to be done. The hospital lawyers, who represented the Board of Trustees, were afraid of what would happen to the hospital if he had another bad case and the medical staff had somehow allowed that to happen. "Do I hear a motion for a summary action?" Immediately there were 40 eyeballs glaring at me, dilated pupils, looks of consternation and fright, and a moment of deafening silence.

"Do you have any idea what he would do to us if we tried that?" Mumbled his internist friend.

A summary action essentially removes a physician from his practice at the hospital if it is feared that he would be of danger to himself, to others, or to his patients. There is a mountain of due process ostensibly protecting the physician so it's not the end of the world. This is where peer review is supposed to make an appearance. As we have learned, peer review is not high on the list of "to-dos" for doctors. Most scrutinized physicians become legal experts and they are deft at waving the wand of antitrust. What was certain was that Nigel would not sit still for a summary action and would not hesitate to take the matter to whatever court. Nigel had made a number of the physicians on the medical executive committee prosperous with his referrals and no one wanted to bite the hand that fed them.

Finally, the chairwoman of the department of anesthesia moved that Nigel be summarily suspended. There were gasps, papers were rattled, and the night air bathed us all in its stifling embrace. From out of nowhere the chairman of pediatrics, a diminutive man, who was assumed by all to be gay, seconded the motion. This was the moment for discussion, but the agenda had worn everyone out. No one said very much so the matter was put to a vote without further discussion. This would be the moment for definitive action. This would be the moment of courage. But, it didn't carry. In fact, nothing more was done. The matter was dropped.

So as I sat in the doctor's dining room, I was privy to this information, but it was protected information, and I ended up mumbling something about the matter was still under review when asked by my colleagues what was going on. But I knew that he had wiggled out of this third bad case. It wasn't long before I heard through the grape vine about a fourth bad case. Most of the pertinent information that came my way did so by this back channel route. With of a dash of insolence, a pinch of daring, and a sprinkle of grandiosity, Nigel had activated his pen and given birth to a fourth bad case. A sensuous smugness filled me. After all it wasn't me whose ass was in the slinger and Nigel was such a prick.

Eventually I learned all of the sordid details.

Fred Stark played third base on the Lions Club softball team. Softball was big in the foothills of the Sierra Nevada. With the same gusto that fueled the early miners of the 19th century, the male residents of the gold country poured their heart and soul into slow pitch softball. Many of these men had played on local high school and Little League baseball teams and this was a way to stay in the game. Third base was a difficult spot, whether it was baseball or softball, being so close to the hitter. Called the hot corner, a third baseman could expect line drives careening off the bat directly towards him at incredible speed. There was less time than the blink of the eye to both defend one's self and to accurately field the ball. Fred still had quick hands, good eye sight, and a strong throw to first base, skills that had helped him become an all star high school third baseman. Even at 60 he was lean and had moves of a much younger man. On hot summer nights he loved to put on his uniform and for just a moment turned back time. These games were usually played before one or two fans, any number of critters -- skunks, raccoons, and porcupines --and those flying and biting creatures called gnats. But it felt good, the smell of leather, the cool night air, the bright lights, and the feel of grass. God, it couldn't get any better.

During the last year or so Fred had began to feel his age, or so he thought. His timing was just a little off, and for a third baseman that could be disaster. He noticed a peculiar numbness in his throwing arm, which he simply attributed to being older and trying to throw harder. But it was hard to understand why his right arm should have a pins and needle feeling. He eventually confided this to his wife and within a short period of time he found himself in the office of his family practice doctor.

Grant Evans had practiced medicine in the gold country for twenty-five years. The community was small and Grant had ministered to nearly every resident at one time or another. He had been an avid softball player himself until an errant throw flew into his face smashing his glasses and nearly leaving him sightless. So, he threw the towel in but his heart remained on the diamond. Fred trusted Grant, who tended to be a little too casual, but had an uncanny ability to smell something wrong. Fred's symptoms bothered Grant. His mind immediately conjured up the story of Lou Gehrig. Grant wasn't absolutely sure but there appeared to be some loss of muscle at the base of Fred's right thumb. That was enough. In an instant he decided to send Fred to Nigel.

Nigel had a very large practice. His reputation thrived in the foothill area and he saw most of the neurological referrals from gold country general practitioners. Nigel's office was imposing. He sat behind a huge mahogany desk. His walls were covered with diplomas. In the corner stood a full human skeleton, not a real one, but the kind you can buy for big bucks and which served partly as decoration, partly as status, and on occasion a way of explaining what was going on to a terrified patient. And Fred was terrified. Nigel changed his pomposity into benevolence. Deep down in his heart he knew that this might be an opportunity to turn his tide of misfortune into brilliance. He yearned for acclaim. With studied concentration he took Fred's history carefully. Before long Fred was whisked into the examining room, which assaulted his senses with its array of diagnostic tools, the overly bright lighting, the fragrance of antisepsis, and the feel of authenticity. Nigel did a very thorough physical exam with particular attention to the neurological exam-- tapping Fred's knees with a percussion hammer, testing his arms for strength and sensation, testing his vision and smell, all the while trying to understand what went on in a softball game. But Nigel was a technophysician, an expert with linear, reductionist curing. What was missing was a soulful reference, that intangible force that comes from a divine-human connection, an understanding that he might not be the best person for the job, that case selection cried out for someone more proficient with the anterior approach, that passing on the case was actually good medicine. Fred was becoming more and more concerned but he also trusted Nigel. Grant had made Nigel into some sort of demi-God and Grant wouldn't steer him wrong.

The technological maze ordered by Nigel led Fred from the imposing CT scanner to the intimidating MRI, to the lab where countless vials of blood were drawn, to cardiology where an EKG was done, to the pulmonary lab where breathing tests were completed. He must have come into contact with thirty different technicians, transporters, clerical persons, nurses and attendants during this journey. All of the equipment was glistening, shiny, imposing, and impersonal. Fred was very alone during these tests, no doctor, no one who seemed to care, no one touched him, the smiles were perfunctory at best and fleeting. The odyssey had been carefully planned, but the various stations at which he stopped seemed disconnected, people often unaware of where he had been, of what had already been done, but overly preoccupied with having him recite the same historical facts about age, allergies, and other illnesses, insurance carrier, family doctor, and, of course, the consent form.

Nevertheless, Fred felt very secure and confident. Like most Americans Fred had come to trust the process if it was blessed by his physician. The marvels of medicine were above reproach. There was a certainty that his best interests were first and foremost. Fred took a "leap of faith" when he placed himself into the CT machine, then the MRI room, then the crown of Medusa, the wires of the EEG. There was no reason to doubt the credibility of any physician. Hadn't they sacrificed so much and spent so much time studying? So what if the process seemed sterile. Fred had always understood that where there was gain there was some pain.

Back in Nigel's office he learned that he had cervical spondylosis. Simply put the bone of his spine had become thicker and was impinging on his spinal cord. At least it was not Lou Gehrig's disease, but serious enough. Not a cancer, not contagious, not a death warrant, but without treatment there would be further compression and eventual paralysis. The conversation was choreografted so that Fred was convinced that paralysis was inevitable without the surgery. No real facts were given. So, Nigel made the decision to operate, to decompress his cervical spine, to prevent total paralysis. Not an unreasonable decision. The procedure would entail a cervical corpectomy, corpus being a Latin word for body, and in this instance removing part of the cervical bone structure to give breathing room to his spinal cord. This could have been done with the safer posterior approach, but it was Nigel's judgment that the more risky anterior approach was warranted. It is likely that a properly trained back surgeon would have chosen the more conservative posterior approach leaving the anterior approach only when it was the only option. This is the essence of proper case selection. Quality dictates what is done. Outcomes are carefully kept in mind. There is no rush to judgment predicated on maintaining or increasing market share, on protecting one's turf, or cashing in on a big-ticket procedure. Orthopedic back surgeons are not immune to economic seduction, but a well trained person generally feels more secure, comfortable with the demands of quality, and would more likely choose the appropriate procedure.

An ad hoc committee was convened because Fred's bad outcome led to another occurrence report. Nurses, physicians doing peer review, or the hospital administrator, generate occurrence reports. This was certainly not Nigel's first such report, but now all of us were getting very nervous about his string of bad cases. Sometimes these occurrence reports were simply handled between the head of whatever department and the subject physician and if there was no merit to it nothing more was done. If it was a fairly minor issue, whether a quality or behavior issue, then a frank discussion might take place between the chief of staff or the head of the physician's department and the involved physician where an opportunity for improvement might be identified. In this case "opportunity for improvement" is a euphemism for "get your shit in order." If it is real bad, like this case, an ad hoc committee is often appointed by the chief of staff to decide whether to proceed with a summary action against the physician. So the ad hoc committee needed to get the facts, to carefully examine the case record and any other pertinent material, to interview the principals including Nigel, and make a recommendation.

The ad hoc committee met in the sixth floor conference room. This was an investigatory committee, ostensibly created to decide what to do about Nigel. Adjacent to the administrator's office and down the hall from the doctor's dining room, we were on neutral ground. The atmosphere was oppressive. The Gods atop Mount Olympus were shaking their fists at us. After all wasn't this one of their own who was being castigated? How dare we meddle in the life of this giant. But there we were, five fairly freaked out medical staff leaders, charged with the unenviable task of confronting Nigel. The was an opportunity for Nigel to help us understand, to explain away this new bothersome case, to help us out of this dilemma. But intuitively I knew that wouldn't be the case. My colleagues were the chief of surgery, the chief of neurosurgery, the chairperson of quality improvement, and the vice chief of staff. Although Nigel was of the opinion that he had no peers, he was also uncomfortable with anyone other than physicians being present. So, the hospital administrator was asked to cool his heels. Another paradox!

We all took our seats and for a moment, which seemed like an eternity, no one spoke a word. We fumbled with our hands, doodled with our pens, those same pens that had the potential to create more of this shit, and gazed furtively out the window. The only noise was the sound of footsteps outside of the conference room. Finally, after a couple of coughs, I explained to Nigel why we were here, as if he didn't know, and what our task was. For the next sixty minutes Nigel lectured to us about subjects ranging from government intervention in medical care to the rigors of a neurosurgical residency. This convoluted, circuitous, self serving monologue approached an end point. With much fear and trepidation, I asked "Nigel, tell us about this Fred Stark business." I had caught him between sentences, between breaths, and now silence again descended and bathed us all in its stillness.

Nigel cleared his throat, wiggled in his chair, straightened up, cocked his head, and looked directly into my eyes, searching for my soul, reaching for the core of my being, and struggling for the high ground answered, "Fred Stark's doing well. He has no problem with my care. We're good friends. I've talked with him on several occasions since he left the rehab hospital and he's satisfied." It was unclear whether any of the committee actually talked to Fred after the operation, but we all saw that he was confined to a wheel chair and rumors were rampant.

Well, that blew us away. That was the sum total of his response. An opportunity for clarity blown away by a heavy dose of ego, all of ours I suppose, but Nigel's ego for sure. We continued on with the deliberation for another hour. We couldn't come to a consensus so we decided to present the issue to the full Medical Executive Committee, that same lethargic committee that looked the other way after the third bad case. No one wanted to take Nigel's job away, no one wanted to risk being sued, no one believed that we could change him, and everyone hoped that this would just blow over. So what was the point of the committee? There was some self satisfaction that we had discharged our duties by fulfilling the bylaws requirement to investigate the possibility that a physician was a danger to himself or others. We got off the hook by throwing it back into the laps of the medical executive committee, even though that committee had not shown any stomach for dealing with the issue. We certainly left the hospital administration and Board of Trustees in a difficult spot if there were another bad case. In the final analysis we simply took care of one of our own, unwilling to face facts, unwilling to risk what was right.

Fred was discharged back to his foothill home. He finally got a chance to return to his beloved softball field where the team was ecstatic to see him again. He actually put on his uniform, which still fit, and the guys played catch with him. It seemed so natural. This sacred ground between the left and right field chalk marks, the grass infield, the dirt at home plate, the firm, anchored bases, base paths that paved the way for America's pastime. If only he could get out of the damn wheelchair, if only he could run out to third base, he would gladly put up with the numbness in his arms for a chance to field a ground ball and throw to first. But, it wasn't to be. Fred would never walk again.

Our astute neurosurgeon, who was overly confident of his abilities and his birth right to carry out the procedure, operated on a lovely man who lived in the foothills, and came for help because he noticed numbness in his throwing arm, making it difficult for him to continue to play on the senior softball team. He was referred to our sanctimonious neurosurgeon, treated to all of his trappings, his supreme confidence, and his questionable reputation. The surgery took forever, in part because this surgeon worked so methodically and slowly, but also because this was new territory for him, albeit he approached the task with bravado. Fred was the ultimate loser.

The MEC is always more invested in protecting a doctor's good name than taking action to either restrict a privilege, or to require more training. The upshot of all their work was to let this guy continue, exposing other patients to the risk of serious complication. Why did it take so long to do something? How could this have happened? In fact, none of the patients injured brought up malpractice issues because of our crusader's charisma, that subjective asset which invites patients to give up their unearned faith and bond with their physician. The MEC eventually put some safeguards in place, but by then, after a lengthy and arduous investigative process, the damage had been done and our neurosurgical whiz had retired.

The real question is how does all of this contribute to escalating health care costs? Isn't this a particular problem, in a particular hospital, and unlikely to represent the overall picture? The amount of money spent to rehabilitate this poor man was abominable, clearly an extra cost, and borne by all of us. This happens every day, across the country with technophysicians, albeit from different disciplines, trying out new and glitzy procedures on unsuspecting patients, with similar results. The combination of lax FDA oversight of medical devices and the cavalier attitude of physicians who take advantage of this situation leads to an environment where technophysicians actually practice on their patients. In small community hospitals, medical staffs and their medical executive committees are generally weak kneed, fearing legal retaliation under the guise of restraint of trade, unwilling to risk friendships and referral sources, and resentful of the fact that they are supposed to deal with these issues.

This is not uplifting information but we patients must beware of it if we are to make informed choices, if we are to take back the night and demand appropriate medical care, if we are to play a meaningful role in dealing with the health care crisis.

Chapter 12
Caduceus: Coming To Understand

The quest for the root cause of the health care crisis continues to oblige me to turn back the pages of my own journey in medicine. The opening salvo of that process was that first day as a medical student, where the whirlwind of activity has required scrutiny. This is the place where the nascent elements of a subconscious awareness of asymmetry in health care began to take form. I am compelled to return to that first day.

Milling in a cavernous hallway with future classmates, mostly men and mostly white, all of us from the top of our respective undergraduate classes, all of us edgy with the knowledge that some of us might not make it, discomfort and uneasiness was replaced by meaningless chatter and nervous handshakes. The smell of apprehension; bodies bumped and pushed; a struggle for breathing room, a search for space to reconnoiter. Perhaps it was the colossal stress we all experienced in those first hours that made lifelong friends of people who would ordinarily not notice one another. A university administrator informed us that from now on this time slot, 8:00 to 10:30, Monday through Friday, would be our class in gross anatomy. Gross anatomy was that time-honored gauntlet, an obstacle to be hurdled early in the process of becoming a doctor. This was where we would learn the ins and outs of Homo sapiens, the circuitry and supporting structures, how we were put together, the proper nomenclature of all the parts we could see with our eyes and hold with our hands. This is where we were to cut our teeth, where we would confront our insecurity, where we take our first steps into the world of health care, into an arena of human suffering. This was the first chapter of learning a new language.

Dr. Patek was our professor. He didn't look particularly happy that day. I would realize later that he never looked happy. He had grown into his subject, as husbands come to look like their wives and owners look like their pets. Dr. Patek, a full professor of anatomy and chair of the department, was a walking, talking cadaver. His waxy, gray face, with its prognathous jaw and acromegalic features have found a lasting place in my mind. His was the course that would make or break a medical student. For weeks we had nervously awaited this most time-honored of medicine's initiations--the anatomy lab. Medical students from Hippocrates to Galen had been denied this privilege, but at that moment that was a concept difficult to appreciate.

With dispassion and method, Dr. Patek introduced gross anatomy. I was petrified. I had seen one or two dead bodies at funerals, where they were carefully positioned in flower-laded coffins, forever at peace and beautifully dressed. The sight of them made me uncomfortable, but flanked by family and friends, I felt myself protected. Now, however, I was to become intimate with a corpse, some unfortunate who had willed his skin, bones and viscera to science, to me and to all of us listening to Dr. Patek. I was all too aware of the thin barrier of fast-disappearing minutes, which rested between me and the corpse that awaited my presence. Gross anatomy meant touching and probing—a complete hands-on experience. There would be no comfort and security of the microscope , where tissues could be inspected behind the safety of a lens. How I longed for that barrier!

A pair of formidable steel doors guarded the anatomy lab, which lay in the basement of the building, directly under the lecture hall. Inside the brilliant light-- sunshine pouring through the ceiling-level windows and buzzing fluorescent-wired overhead blinded us. Noises echoed with thumps and clatters as we arranged ourselves in groups of four to behold our cadavers--twenty-five such creatures wrapped in plastic on cold steel gurneys, heads positioned northward. Next to our corpse laid the instruments of torture--our dissecting tools. I felt a rustling of my starched white coat. Beside me were three similarly clad students who would constitute the lab group I would belong to. This was the formal organization that the university rather arbitrarily created. Our long white coats served to protect our clothes from the slippery, putrid formaldehyde. The smell would cease to affect us in a matter of days. We donned our white coats before descending the steps to the other side of the River Styx. They were brand-new, gleaming and full-length, the kind worn by doctors in the movies and real doctors who worked in hospitals. A caduceus, the symbol of medicine, was embroidered above the right pocket: the ancient staff of Hermes entwined by a pair of snakes. At the top were wings. When I fastened the buttons, the coat reached nearly to the floor. This was my military uniform, a suit of armor, a badge of courage. It would tell the outside world that I was a medical student, nearly a doctor. We were all being knighted, though we hadn't earned our right of passage yet.

I named our cadaver Matilda. It seemed then and now to be terribly irreverent, but gallows humor has a way of prevailing and for no explainable reason the name stuck. Matilda had apparently died of a type of lymphoproliferative disease-- leukemia or lymphoma-- and death's signature was a series of lumps at the base of her neck, in her armpits and groin, and a distended abdomen from an enlarged liver and spleen. Though dead, she no longer looked human. It was evident that she had once been a person, but the idea seemed incredibly abstract. Slippery and stinking, she was a product of hundreds of thousands of years of evolution, the most complex species that life had to offer, a person like me from the 20th century--someone's mother, maybe a waitress, a secretary or a lawyer. But she was missing anima, soul, intelligence, language, movement, warmth and another element--that something spiritual that ties us all to a source of universal power, maybe God.

It is this intangible element that has so engaged me over the years. How can it be that a person suffers so much, with fatigue, pain, or nausea and the affected body part cannot be identified? I believe that with chronic illness, or at least many chronic illnesses, human beings suffer because of a dislocation of their souls, a separation from our higher power or whatever celestial entity that loves and protects us. This is not something dissectible from our cadavers. I didn't learn this in my gross anatomy or histology classes. From a physical or anatomical point of view, we are all put together amazingly similarly. Any class in gross anatomy will prove that. But there is something to each of us, some life force that works differently from one person to the next, that makes us individually vulnerable, susceptible in our own unique way to hardship and the vicissitudes of life; a life force which helps us reach out of this abyss of nothingness to create meaning. If all we had to do was review our notes from anatomy, pathology and biochemistry, it would be easier to be a good doctor. Neither gross anatomy nor Gray's *Anatomy*, the text that every medical student underlines compulsively, could teach me a thing about this cosmic force that had once been part of Matilda, the energy that pulses through a living human being, that makes her who she is and distinguishes her from each and every one of her collective brothers and sisters. Matilda was to offer up many mysteries, but never a clue to the woman she had once been. I could only wonder.

We were chained to her, for she was the requisite launching point of our ambitions and dreams. To succeed meant to study Matilda. We were motivated, committed, even altruistic in seeing healing as our direction. Very few of us viewed it as a strategy, an investment of ourselves, a road of financial transactions. This was a period of purity in our lives. Our motives were honest, our vision the measure of our dedication, our resolve fueled by the passion of helping others. We bonded to each other immediately--a very human way to deal with overwhelming stress. Not one of our other courses--histology, physiology or biochemistry--presented the juice and essence we found in the guts of Matilda, laid bare in the bright white light of the anatomy lab. It was on her sinews that we would cut our teeth, it was she who would know our insecurity, and it was with her that we would take our first steps into the word of health care, into the arena of human suffering.

Her lifelessness aside, Matilda and I developed a relationship. She was a discrete and familiar form, a particular and distinct individual. From the time we parted to a point much later in my career, the lines between my patients would blur. The patients I was assigned in medical school, those I tended during my training years, and those I saw in private practice were all much less distinct to me, part of a large and amorphous group of individuals to whom I related in terms of their symptoms and diagnoses. The more successful I became, the more financial gains that were available, the harder I worked and the more patients I saw, the more willing I grew to overlook their individuality in my quest for success, the more difficult it was to return to the lessons I learned from Matilda. At that time in my life I abandoned the search for the intangible element. I was blind to the life force I had wondered about in the months I had explored Matilda. The more I whirled with the world of medicine, the world of *scientific* medicine, the easier it was to ignore those wonderings. The road marks of science were so well laid out and so easy to see. They were profitable and tangible.

It would be many years before I once again became aware of the most important information Matilda had given me. What remains indelibly imprinted in my memory is the caduceus embroidered on my new white coat. It wasn't long before the coat was so soiled that it ended up in the round file. But that Caduceus!! Here was a symbol, which included a short rod entwined by two snakes and topped by a pair of wings. The caduceus was the magic wand of the Greek god Hermes (Roman Mercury), messenger of the gods, inventor of magical incantations, conductor of the dead and protector of merchants and thieves. Many medical organizations use this symbol and it shouldn't have been a surprise to find it on my coat. As the myth goes the snakes were found copulating and forcibly separated by Tiresias—the seer who was so unhelpful to Oedipus and his family. For that he was turned into a woman, and remained so for seven years, until he was able to repeat his action and change back to a male. The transformative power in this story, strong enough to completely reverse even physical polarities of male and female, comes from the union of the two serpents, passed on by the wand. There was symmetry in this symbol: a precarious balance between the staff and snakes; the two snakes, one staff, and at the top a pair of wings. What did the wings mean? Was flight possible only when the staff and snakes were balanced, harmonious, integrated, and symmetrical?

****

It was several years later when I met Rose Silverman. I was still totally involved in my lengthy and arduous training program and I was starting to feel good about myself. Rose Silverman was a native born Angeleno. Early in the century her parents moved to Hollywood where her father had been a movie producer of modest success. Rose met Saul Silverman at UCLA and they were married shortly after graduation. Saul had become a wealthy financier and together they had enjoyed a privileged life. When I first saw Rose, she had been a widow for ten years. This octogenarian was the matron of a large family, many of whom were professionals, all of whom continued to live in Los Angeles. Five years previously her children persuaded Rose to move to an upscale residential home. Her eyesight was failing, she had fallen and broken a hip just before the move, and in spite of her caring family, she was lonely and a little depressed. The residential home was a godsend. Rose met several other ladies with similar backgrounds and her outlook brightened considerably. She was still able to participate in family get togethers, outings to the Temple, vacations and celebrations. She retained her keen wit, her nimble linguistic skills, interspersing Yiddish with English at the most outlandish moments. Simple conversation became hilarity at a moment's notice. She could be a total nut. She had become a sage, a moral pillar, a source of strength and healing to her family. She was a wealthy woman and she did not hesitate wearing expensive clothes and jewelry, but at her core, there resided a spark of humility.

On a non-descript foggy March morning, Rose called her eldest son to tell him she was having trouble breathing. He drove right over, only to find his mother as blue gray as her hair, and so breathless that she could not complete a sentence. He immediately put her into his car, not certain what he should do, and drove to the largest hospital he could find, which happened to be Los Angeles County General Hospital. I am not sure if this is what he had in mind, but that's where they ended up, that's where Rose was hospitalized. It didn't take long for the resident on call to spot congestive heart failure and Rose was promptly admitted to the ICU. Within an hour, several other family members had arrived, terribly concerned and waiting expectantly in a room just off the ICU. Rose had been given medication, and breathing more easily, had perked up. Soon, with her purse in her hand, she was demanding to go home. The cardiologist on call told her she had had a heart attack and was not going home just yet. Rose was not happy.

I was paged and asked me to see Mrs. Silverman in consultation ASAP. I immediately went to the ICU where Rose was bent over an emesis basin filled with dark blood. The sight of this frail, breathless, woman, vomiting blood, becoming weaker, stamped a sense of urgency on the situation. The bleeding had begun on her second hospital day and her hemoglobin had fallen precipitously. The first of two units of blood had been started and her vital signs were now stable. The vomiting slowed considerably after the nurses inserted a nasogastric tube. This large bore tube insured some order to the chaos, the blood was now removed from her stomach in an orderly fashion, without the hideous vomiting, by way of a suction device attached to the wall. Yet, the price Rose paid was the discomfort this imposing plastic device caused, invading her body through one nostril, adding disfigurement to her pain. In the intensive care unit her face was covered with an oxygen mask, her hands immobilized by intravenous catheters in both arms, there was a central venous catheter under her right clavicle. Rose looked like a helpless caged animal, fighting for control, fighting to establish her territory, to protect her space, to guard her humanness.

Rose's family wanted everything done. No one had taken the time or effort to share with the family her guarded prognosis. No one had actually told Rose how grave her situation was. No one had discussed with her the impact a "full court press" might have on her quality of her life. No one had actually made her a partner in her own health care. I had the sense that the ICU nurses were frustrated by the situation, that all our ministrations and enthusiasm might not be appropriate, that what we were doing might be an assault on Rose's dignity. But what did the nurses know? We were the ones who were the recipients of the legacy of medical science achievements. We were the anointed ones who would apply the fruits of the latest research, the refinements of he latest techniques, the wonder of modern medicine to rescue the doomed patient. Rose was unable to speak. I got a rough sketch of what was going on from the family, and, within a short period of time I learned a great deal about her life. The family was pleading for some direction, holding hands, weeping, at times angry, and at times, saddened. A cursory physical exam and a brief review of lab data left me pondering what to do.

I remember her eyes. They were beautiful, mournful, laden with the memory of other, now distant, trials, tribulations, and pain. There was a touch of serenity, but this was accented by defiance, a will to overcome, a will to live. She couldn't move, couldn't talk, could communicate very little, but she was in the moment, gathering her strength, harvesting her wits, calculating, ready for what was to come. I was uneasy. Jesus, the nurses made me uneasy. The faith that the family had already invested in my capabilities unnerved me. The whole situation was uncomfortable.

For just a brief moment I wondered about the right thing to do, but how could a trainee in a large academic medical center decline to carry out a procedure that had been requested by another physician-in-training who was backed by his faculty person. As a house officer, another term for an intern, resident, or fellow, we are taught by example, how our professors approach a certain problem. When faculty writes an opinion regarding the diagnosis and treatment on a particular chart, that is sacrosanct. The wise house officer does not complain or upset the cookie jar, he does what the faculty suggested. The whole goddamn medical educational system required that doctors not rebel, success was predicated on conformity, doing it like it had been done, not rocking the boat. Deep down I had the feeling that an invasive test might be unnecessary, that it wouldn't make any overall difference in her care, but these were just fleeting, ill defined, thoughts. It was as if my basic sense of propriety had been shifted, my take on the human condition adulterated, my connection to the quality of life severed. It was all too easy to assuage one's self with the notion that sanctity of life was preeminent, that life was so precious, so sacred, that any effort or measure to preserve it, even if it might not actually be recognized as "life" after medical intervention, was justified.

There I was, poised with my scope, my probe, protecting me from her misery, a buffer between me and this dying patient, and cheered on by the family, the faculty, all who had placed their faith in this physical science paradigm. As if I could control events with this scope, as if any of us could control events, as if we could change the course of destiny. Yet, could we? There was now a large part of me that actually believed that I was in control and that by virtue of my own self will I could change in a meaningful and significant way the course of events for this woman.

So I scoped her. Rose wasn't able to sign a consent form but I explained the procedure in a fashion. I did not tell her that this would be one more assault on her dignity; that if gentle sedation did not suffice, her health care team, me, the nurses, the orderlies and aids, were prepared to use force to get our way; that her family, who had provided the surrogate approval, would not be with her. I could see those questions in her eyes but I tried to comfort myself that she knew even less than the nurses about this marvelous technology.

The battle began with conscious sedation. Because her heart was in a weakened condition, I decided that less that the usual amount of Demerol and Valium was to be given intravenously. She watched expectantly as I slowly gave the medicine. She fought back, refusing to surrender, refusing to abandon her senses, eyes defiant and wide open. We sprayed her throat with a local anesthetic, she was unwilling to open her lips which still had bright red lipstick at the corners; the tiny administration tube was forced towards the back of her throat and the medicine dispensed as an aerosol. She coughed, grimaced, spit it out and forced her body to writhe, twist and turn. A dance of defiance, she willed a controlled spasm, fighting as best she could, with limited control and few options. In retrospect, it was clear to me that she had not given consent, even though a perfunctory one was given. I believe she felt trapped; she knew what her family wanted, but this clashed with her own will. She was not demented, she was caught in a paradox.

When we felt that she was adequately sedated, she was forced onto her left side. Her tubes became tangled causing us some consternation. I detected a faint smile on her face; all the while we were encouraging her, pleading with her to understand how important this test was, how easy it would be, how quickly it would be over. She shook her head back and forth, she made it very difficult for us to straighten out and preserve the attachments of all of her supporting tubes and wires. We substituted a prong-type nasal cannula for her facemask to continue the flow of oxygen.

From the corner of her eyes she could see the long black snake; that marvelous technological advancement called a gastroscope; a tightly bound bundle of fiber optics, a sinister life form which could bend at its tip to the right or left, up or down, by virtue of the control knob in my hands. The diameter of the scope was not more than one inch but the impact of the thing depends which end of the scope you are facing. We continued to plead, to cajole, to bark orders:-- "keep your head down, breath quietly through you nose, the oxygen will protect you, try not to gag, swallow only when I say , then relax and let your saliva drool out your mouth so we can suction it." She would not flex her neck, she kept her head in an erect position, daring us to force it down, inviting us to join the fray. So we did. The hefty orderly grasped her legs, held them together, immobilized, while the guy at the head of the bed forced her head to the pillow and forced it to flex. Her bed clothes were thrown asunder, she was now naked before the world, a frail body, sagging flesh, protuberant bones and joints, unsightly varicosities, moles, scars, her persona betrayed.

Where was the faculty that wanted the fucking test? What would her family think if they had been there? Where on the consent form was what we were doing? As an afterthought the nurses tried to remove her dentures. She clinched her teeth with all of her energy, generating a considerable force which nature has supplied all carnivorous mammals, compelling me to use a tongue blade which was threaded between her dentures and made to touch the back of her throat causing an involuntary gag and opening of her mouth.

At just the right moment the padded middle part of the tongue blade, designed for seizure patients to prevent them from biting their tongues, was turned on its side to force her mouth further open. The nurse then slipped her fingers into her mouth and dislodged her dentures, protected by the padded tongue blade. The trauma from this endeavor caused her gums to bleed and added a surreal dimension to the battle. With her head forced down, her dentures pulled free, her legs held tightly, the moment of truth was at hand.

By now I was angry. Why is she making this so difficult? Why are we doing this to her? How can she be so sick and so strong? Why doesn't she just let us do our job? I picked up the scope with both hands. My left hand held the control knobs, the suction and insufflation buttons (reminding me of a trumpet), and my right hand handled he leading end of the scope, the part that would pass through her lips and mouth into her esophagus and then into her stomach. I carefully lubricated this end of the instrument and began to insert it. She became enraged, straining, yelling, screaming, thrashing. She lost control of her bowels; the bedclothes now soiled with malodorous stool admixed with old blood.

We debated giving more sedation but would her heart take it? I decided it would not. By now it had become a battle of two wills, hers and mine. My faculty adviser, my teacher, was detained and so I was on my own, something that had happened before and was ok since I had already had "enough experience." I became less a doctor than a wrestler and I gave free reign to my sub cortical instincts. I handed the control end of the instrument to the nurse and with both hands pried open her mouth, securing the scope into the back of her mouth, keeping it in middle, slightly flexed and in position as she gagged, screamed, and spit. After a few interminable seconds she involuntarily swallowed, which allowed the scope to slide into her esophagus. During this period of time her blood oxygen fell to dangerous levels in spite of the nasal oxygen and in part because she was holding her breath. When the scope passed into her esophagus there was a brief moment of retreat, rather, a moment of respite, a chance for her to reorganize, reconnoiter, and gather strength with her second wind. But, by now I was more fully in control.

The beautifully designed instrument was performing like a ballerina, dancing here and there at my touch, and relaying clear images through the eyepiece by way of the thousands of fiber optic glass strands. There were still some residual blood clots in the dependent part of her stomach, but not obscuring the view of an ulcer seen at the end of her stomach. So, she had an ulcer, which was not bleeding, which had a firm adherent clot, and the ulcer appeared benign. She fought throughout the procedure. We had more clinical information, everyone, except Rose, seemed satisfied. I was relieved. She actually survived that procedure. One of the wonders of conscious sedation is that the patient is amnesic for the event, a blessing for both of us. I wondered how I had helped. Her family thanked me profusely for which I was grateful, my ego was stroked, a potent intoxicating tonic, but there were still vestiges of doubt about what I had done. Maybe I was so anxious for approval that it was too hard to resist these accolades.

Shortly after the procedure Rose had a stroke. I do not believe it was related to the procedure, but rather the bleeding and anemia. But in my heart it was debatable. Her right side was now paralyzed, her mouth drooped, spittle dripped from her lips, she could no longer talk or laugh. I saw her one or two times after the debacle but the visits were perfunctory and obligatory. Within a short period of time she was transferred to another part of the hospital called telemetry where her heart rhythm could be closely monitored. I didn't see her again, but I learned that she was unable to return to her residential home. Instead, she was transferred to a nursing home. She was no longer able to continue to participate in the celebratory events of her family. She was unable to travel much further than the lanai of the nursing home. Going for drives and going to parties were out of the question. The more I learned of her plight, the more reluctant I was to visit her. Besides, our job was finished. We specialists had done what we were trained to do. The outcome was not good, but we did what had to be done. Or did it have to be done?

What was it about Rose? There was a clear cut relationship between her defiance and willful choice and Hemmingway's fish. Rose pissed me off because she was on moral high ground and I was on a slippery slope. Rose carried lessons she had learned from the holocaust, lessons about choice, about defiance, about staking a claim. If she had been made part of the decision making process, if she were allowed to express her own take of the situation, her feelings about what we wanted to do, it may have led to a more conservative approach, which in this case likely would have been a better choice. In emergencies, we sometimes do things that patients would not approve of, but in that situation the patient is usually unconscious, demented, or unable to communicate. In her case, she was able to communicate by virtue of the struggle, but we were convinced that we had all of the answers because we were blessed by the university, the faculty, and this citadel of training. She became a benchmark for me, a reminder of the strength that flows from doing the right thing, something that requires meaningful communication with he patient who is in possession of that intangible life force.

There would be other instances in the future when I had convinced myself that a procedure had helped my patient, but deep down there was always doubt. There were times when I was certain when endoscopy helped to make a diagnosis, and later, when there were more therapeutic options available, I felt even more comfortable that I had made a difference, but so many times I wondered. On so many occasions it was hard to justify what I had done, how the procedure helped the suffering patient, how this probe contributed to healing. Sure she survived. But, maybe she would have survived whether or not she was assaulted by the gastroscope. We have come to understand that most people do survive this type of bleed, and clinical research has been directed at identifying those most likely to continue bleeding, or to rebleed. But sometimes it's a crapshoot. And, what have we accomplished?

Why do we technophysicians do this? Because we can. The system has blessed us with a carte blanche, a not-so benevolent approval, and we patients have co-signed the whole thing. Do we technophysicians do these things because we actually believe that the outcomes justify the ordeal? Sometimes, but more often than not, there are other perfidious motivations at work. The system itself is calcified, unable to remold itself, unable to close the yawning gap between science and technology, satisfied that technology is inherently the right answer. The medical educational system invites students to follow without question the advice and recommendations of teachers, instilling a herd mentality, and leaving the new technophysician with precious little objectivity in deciding who should or should not have a procedure. This coupled with the monetary rewards paves the way for unscrupulous technophysicians who are busy contributing mightily to the ever-increasing rise in health care expenditures.

Technophysicians are so wrapped up in completing the procedure successfully that they not infrequently expose the patient to harm, oblivious to fragile vital signs, which may become an issue during a difficult and prolonged procedure. Technophysicians plod on, committed to completing the surgery or procedure, even when the patient is doing poorly. By now, towards the end of my training in gastroenterology, it was clear that caducean asymmetry had something to do with health care maladies. This jump to high technology violates the symmetry of the caduceus. The Staff of Hermes, that messenger of high technology, insures an overly masculine approach to illness. When the mythological snakes, representing the feminine side, are properly coiled around the staff of Hermes, harmony is achieved. The feminine side of the equation speaks to the intuitive part, inviting physicians to become healers, employing touch, feeling, and empathy. These elements soften the edges of science, balancing cure with healing. Healing is given its due, illness is differentiated from disease, and the linear, reductionist methodology is removed from its top billing on the marque making room for holism. Medicine's challenge is to integrate mind, body, and spirit.

Hippocratic healing was focused on "dis-ease" rather than diseases understood as ontological entities or perturbations of the universe's machinery that God somehow set into action. This was clearly pre-Greek, pre Scholastic, and pre-Cartesian thinking, but it preserved the whole, including both the bodily and spiritual dimensions of humanness. Hippocratic medicine was bedside medicine. Physicians watched, waited, talked with their patients, won their trust, and gave a helping hand to the "healing power of nature." A fragile detente won't do. All three are important. Healing into wholeness is about all three.

On that warm spring day when I graduated from medical school I was scarcely aware of the importance of the Hippocratic oath. At best a grouping of arcane words, the real meaning didn't sink home until I came to understand how flawed the masculine-only approach is. It takes a balanced male-female approach to have any impact on healing. We are creatures of God, not a sophisticated bundle of circuitry on automatic pilot, not a dualistic separation of mind and body, not simply intellect, psyche and soma, but beings with a spiritual dimension, a spark of divinity in each of us, with a meaningful connection to a universal power who some call God. We are in control of our own square yard of the universe, but nothing more. In spite of our struggles with the realities of life, the universe operates independent of what we think or do. When we are distraught, when we suffer, it is incumbent to first take inventory of ourselves rather than try and change the universe. We need to accept life on life's terms and not waste our time trying to reorder the cosmos. There is a difference between acceptance and approval. We see deceit and dishonesty on a daily basis, but it is what it is, it must be accepted as such, but it does not deserve our approval. This is the way to change, paying attention to our own square yard of the universe first and foremost and making use of the power that flows from a celestial connection. Developing a relationship with that higher power, solidifying the divine- human connection is healthy. When we fight against the universe, this is where illness is born. We are free to follow our own free-will but we run the risk of dislocation between ourselves and this universal power. The result is illness.

The pathway from Matilda to Rose made me more aware of how holism and the metaphysical experience impacted healing. I came to believe that caducean symmetry did not require the elimination of the scientific method or medical technology, any more than healing required a commitment to spiritualism at the expense of high technology. The lingering question was why the asymmetry and how did this contribute to the health care crisis?

Chapter 13
Dr. Young's Ointment: The Managed Care Folly

The political solution to the health care crisis will inevitably be some sort of managed care. What the government can do is to redistribute and reallocate funds in a way that all Americans receive health care. But, what kind of health care? With the recent passage of the Obama health care package the political winds are now blowing in the direction of federally required and subsidized insurance coverage.

Managed care is a broad term and has come to include several elements including an integrated multispecialty health care delivery system, often bonded in some way to a hospital, and prospective payment system to physicians who are salaried rather than on the traditional fee-for service basis. There are different variations of this approach including the Kaiser model, the staff model, as illustrated by the Harvard Community Health Plan employing salaried physicians, or the group model, which is an exclusive arrangement between the payer and a group of physicians.

The newest version envisioned in the recent Obama ACA (Affordable Healthcare Act) is an Accountable Care Organization, which will essentially return us to the managed care format. The expectation is that quality will be served when groups of physicians representing different specialties participate, offering their individual expertise, committed to quality as determined by science, the utilization of electronic medical records, a commitment to control costs, and a willingness to forgo the traditional fee-for-service format. The ACO concept includes a connection with a hospital, with the manager being the hospital or groups of physicians.

But it is in fact a return to the dear old managed care format that was so disliked during the 1990s.

At present there are about 100 of these integrated health care delivery systems including Kaiser, the Mayo clinic and the Geisinger Health System and there is some evidence that that integrated care is positively correlated with improved quality. However, many, if not most physicians are not in groups and a major challenge is to reformulate physician practices in such a way that they are integrated with hospitals and willing to accept salaries that are essentially doled out by the government. This is the rub and a major obstacle to reformulation of health care in America. It is certainly true that many physicians, especially technophysicians, are focused upon making more money. But quality based physicians appreciate the opportunity to make more money predicated upon their mastery of quality. And, why not? Being rewarded for effort and quality is at the heart of capitalism.

When managed care was tried in the 1990s is was not successful when contracting with small groups of physicians and individual doctors. Part of the problem was the heavy handed management of the composition of these groups, regulating the number and types of physician specialists, the availability and regulation of diagnostic tests, surgeries, procedures, hospitalizations and pharmaceuticals. The payers were often for profit HMOs whose primary allegiance was to the stockholders, with little interest and care regarding quality. The payers under Obama care will include the government, with the same heavy-handed management. Heavy-handed management is a poor substitute for meaningful physician involvement, involvement that includes practicing quality medicine and being open to a divine-human connection. But, if technophysicians continue to have their way, driving up expenditures, they will open the doors to extraneous control.

As we have seen, quality continues to be in need of definition, a job that physicians must do but are often not interested in doing, and thus a weak spot. What needs to be understood is how this will play out if the federal government becomes the payer. The government or its proxy will most assuredly be invested with making clinical decisions that adversely affect outcomes, lessons learned in the 1990's with for profit HMOs, because government will hold the purse strings. The largest payer, which will be the government, will most likely micromanage health care decisions, approve and decline procedures on the basis of cost, and undermine the patient-physician relationship. Many of the managed care organizations of the 1990s were not successful because of decisions that emphasized retained earnings only, leaving both the providers and patient dissatisfied. Government hired physicians will play a major role in managing cost from an administrative point of view, where the mission of healing will necessarily will be obfuscated by the government's need to control costs. I believe that health care is a fundamental right and not a privilege, but the methodology of achieving this goal may well throw the baby out with the wash.

I believe that most of the administrative tasks will primarily fall to lay persons. It should seem quite obvious that this system will be problematic because health care engineers can only control costs, not improve quality. Physicians hired by government to participate in these administrative tasks will necessarily trade in their stethoscopes for a pen striped suit, reflecting the need to control costs as a condition of staying employed by the government and at the same time forced to abandon whatever healing instincts they have. The problem is not technomedicine per se, but rather technophysicians who bastardize technomedicine for their own well being. Thus, the government's approach will most likely be a shotgun approach, decimating all layers of the delivery system, including well intentioned and motivated physicians, in an effort to eliminate technophysicians.

The most effective integrated health care delivery systems have been those attached to major tertiary teaching centers. Mayo is a good example. There is no question but that quality is well served here where the system is blessed with talented teachers and scientific researchers. Physicians who are lucky enough to obtain advanced training at Mayo readily accept salaries and quality management, which is traded for a robust education. This would not be the case when today's private physicians are rounded up and forced into an integrated group practice. I have seen how this works and it is not a happy picture.

Nobody seems happy and even the costs have not been controlled. The failure to reduce expenditures during the 1990s when managed care was king is persuasive evidence. The focus is necessarily to see patients in a conveyer belt fashion, because of time constraints, and restricting expensive services with an eye towards cost control rather than quality. Again, if the task is to simply fund technomedicine 'more carefully', then all physicians, which includes quality based physicians, would be punished, rather than focus on the rehabilitation of technophysicians. The task of rehabilitation would best done by physicians, not "providers", who understand the notion of healing; but I believe that government sponsored health care engineers would see this process as inefficient and time consuming. Given the crisis discussed above and the government's interest in solving it, there is a need to understand what it would be like to have government sponsored health care.

Life not only imitates art, but it ruffles the sensibilities of ordinary men with its audacious quirks. Managed care was born of the politics of Richard Milhouse Nixon; it was during his administration that the concept of Health Maintenance Organizations took form. These were essentially insurance companies that purported to manage the care of their patients in a way that was more controlled than with the fee-for-service methodology. The receipt of federal development funds in exchange for mandated market access was part of the deal. This innocuous piece of legislation gained momentum and sent shock waves through the medical establishment. In the midst of Watergate and Vietnam, rising health care costs incredibly caught the attention of an administration under siege from all sides, an administration hurdling pell mell into inferno; and, somehow, in the midst of this turmoil, political changes, which included managed care, swept across the land prefacing a new economic reality for health care.

The notion is fairly simple: The way to control spiraling costs is to put the industry on a budget; physicians or physician groups were given a sum of money by HMOs to cover the medical costs of a group of subscriber/patients during a set period of time; any costs exceeding this lump sum during this time period would be borne by the doctors. Physicians would think twice before ordering expensive tests and patients would be better served by attention to preventive measures and quality care. It was a method to control the costs and complexity of health care. It was a directive to harness the rising health care costs and reformulate a system of payment, which seemed to create a conflict of interest for physicians. In actual fact, managed care has created another conflict of interest for physicians who have been rewarded for doing less and keeping costs down so that money would be left over and distributed amongst themselves. Such a simple concept. Yet, managed care has disrupted the easy ebb and flow between physicians, their patients, and the insurance companies. In the early years it appeared to work. In the 1990s the rising cost of health care, which was rising at 8 to 10% per year, was reduced to 2 to 3%, presumably by managed care. This honeymoon period was soon over, and the rate of increase of health care returned to previous values toward the end of this decade. Part of this was due to inflation, part due to the rising costs of technology, drugs and labor, but we must not lose sight of the power of the pen. It was immediately clear that greed permeated the interstices of not only the health care providers, but also the insurance companies, or HMOs, as well. Some of the earlier not-for-profit plans attempted to provide health care in a more rational and affordable manner. However, armed with new power and the premiums of a large number of takers, the reformulated insurance industry, abandoning their non profit status, made a bundle through new heavy handed contracts with groups of doctors. Flush with success, they had their way with physicians; now the authors of draconian contracts; at the same time assuming for themselves the role of provider by virtue of approving and disapproving tests and treatments; micromanaging the composition of physician groups by eliminating over-represented specialties, eliminating high cost specialties, changing the role of general physicians into gate-keepers who became traffic cops deciding whether, when, and where a patient would be sent on to a specialist. A much better plan would include physicians in all aspects of the decision making process, physicians who understand that technophysicians are the problem and this problem must be dealt with.

The birth of managed care signaled a tumultuous redirection of health care; the avarice and prodigality of the fee-for-service system was replaced by insensitivity, mediocrity, and a struggle between the HMOs, the hospitals, and the government for the power of the physician's pen. That Holy Grail was now the major spoil sought after by these three combatants. The perfidious invaders fought over the booty once the walls erected by the AMA were breached. The landscape changed: a systemic approach to the practice of medicine evolved; the patient physician encounter began to fade from focus. On any given day physicians can expect to see hostile patients, patients who are convinced that managed care is simply a means to enhance profits, patients who are accustomed to more personal care, patients who would rather do battle with a clerk or a real live voice on the telephone. Given the perfidious nature of managed care, these reactions are understandable. These hostile patients seem to come out of nowhere, no warning, only a cog in the otherwise well oiled machinery of day to day practice. Managed care has given new meaning to the word hostility. It seems to be the rule, rather than the exception, that at least one hostile patient will be seen per day. It can happen in the office or in the hospital; it really doesn't matter. Hostility and unhappy patients certainly happened before managed care, but the very nature of this insensitive system has in my opinion led to an exponential increase in their numbers.

****

Eric Sweeny was a general surgeon whose office was next to mine, at a time when I was part of an integrated health care delivery system in Sacramento, which had contracted with several different HMOs and was bonded with a north area hospital. Although somewhat diminutive and short in stature, his surgical skills more than made up for his peculiar physiognomy, and translated him into a giant of a man. He was very particular, somewhat devoid of charisma, but caring and to the point. He relished the opportunity to tell me the following story:

It was on a fairly ordinary day when he had his first combat experience with Letha Simmons. Letha was the prototypical pissed off patient who was fed up with the nuisances of managed care. To Letha the only good thing about managed care was the affordable premiums. She didn't like the idea of being restricted to doctors that she hadn't chosen herself. She didn't like the suspicions that androids were making her appointments. She didn't like the feeling that she was on a conveyer belt. She was divorced and hated men. There didn't appear to be an ounce of levity in her demeanor. She wore plain black pants, with a plaid shirt, and Berkenstock sandals: no perfume, no makeup, no jewelry, just a scowl. The referring physician's expectation was that Eric would help with her diagnosis of pruritus ani, in essence an itchy anus. Her referring doctor thought pruritus ani might be a surgical problem, which really didn't help Eric's mood, because Eric understood more clearly than the referring doctor that this was not a surgical problem. Since he was a general surgeon, his task was to plan if and when to operate, and since surgery was out of the question, he saw this as a waste of his time. He continued with the story.

After an examination of this delicate part of her anatomy, Eric straightened up and said, "Mrs. Simmons, this is not a surgical case and your doctor shouldn't have sent you here."

When groups of doctors band together in managed care to work out the best contract with different HMOs, primary care providers become gate-keepers, essentially directing patients to whatever specialist thought to be appropriate. The opening salvo of a pitched battle begins when the patient demands to be sent to a particular specialist. This has changed somewhat; today some HMOs allow patients to go directly to the specialist they choose. Patients have become accustomed to seeing specialists early on. There is a general consensus that primary care physicians in an HMO-driven physician group are not to be trusted. Recall my consternation with the educational development of this new breed of primary care physician during the period when I was active at UC Davis Medical School. They have perfected the art of "buff and turf" in part because they have a limited time with each patient because of the constraints of cost control. Often finding himself unable to cope with a demanding patient, the poor guy hoists a white flag, and gives in, sending the now infuriated patient to the specialist of choice. In the heat of battle, mistakes are often made and the wrong type of specialist may be chosen. Then, there is the maze of bureaucracy, the time delay for the specialist's appointment, and so, voila, the ingredients for rage.

Letha kicked off her paper gown, sat stark naked, and shook her finger at Eric.

"Why are you putting me off?"

"I'm not putting you off. I'm just trying to tell you that you're in the wrong place." He did try to explain to her that her treatment would not require surgery, but by now Letha was not pleased, to say the least.

"There's no right place here", Letha snarled. "This place is just a maze, a mad house, with idiots at every stop."

Eric now tried to stand a little taller and replied, "If you're calling me an idiot I don't appreciate that. Furthermore, there's not much else I can do for you."

Letha retorted, "Well, right now you're here and I want something done."

Eric shared with me that many expletives rolled around in his mind, but he thought better of biting back. "Okay. There is a special ointment that I can prescribe for you. A colleague of mine concocted it for this type of problem. It's called Dr. Young's Anal Ointment." He went on to explain how to apply it, what to expect, and that there were no side effects. Letha cocked her head just slightly, redressed herself with the paper covering, grunted, cleared her throat, and said, "I'll try it."

I heard about the final chapter of this whole fiasco several weeks later when Eric came rushing into my office. "Hansen, you won't believe what I got in the mail." With Eric most anything was possible. For a split second I tried to imagine what he was talking about; but, for only a split second. With a touch of sardonic humor I responded, "Please tell me what you got."

The denouement went something like this: With his face breaking into a childlike smile he said, *"a piece of ass."* Now I've shared a lot of dirty jokes with the guy, but this was ridiculous. I naturally had to ask him to explain, although part of me really didn't want to know. The insatiable curious part of me won out and I heard the rest of the story.

Eric went on to explain how Letha Simmons took a piece of desquamated anal tissue, simply harvesting her own encrusted anal tissue, and enclosed it in a greeting card that read, "Up yours."

It was obvious that she wasn't happy with this entire ordeal, but there was more to it than that. What was clear was that this patient, like so many others I've dealt with since the onset of managed care, had the audacity to relate to her physician in a very condescending and irreverent manner. Patients clearly have a roll to play in the direction of their care, but inappropriate behavior is no more appropriate for the patient than for the physician. The integrity of the physician/patient encounter was assaulted. Physicians are not entitled to veneration, but desultory animosity like this suggests that managed care patients are outraged with the system. Sure, Eric could have handled things differently, his attitude may have been part of the problem, but it appears to me that rage was present long before she initially saw him; what I heard from Eric was that she was ready to fight before they shook hands.

I believe that patients like this one are firing without aim; a shotgun approach born of the system's inattention and disrespect. We doctors are often seen as representatives of the health care system. It was certainly possible that Letha's ire was solely directed to Eric and his attitude, since she did send the tissue to him. But I have often seen how managed care has raised patient dissatisfaction to the level of fury, holding the physician responsible for the broken system. I've certainly had patients become angry with me, but if I looked closely I could sometimes identify something I had done or not done to provoke the outburst. If I was savvy, I could usually control the situation and prevent this sort of thing from getting out of hand. But, with managed care, patients are sensitized by the system; by the time they get to me there is not much to be done. There is no readily available anecdote to diffuse the situation. Managed care has led to an inexorable transformation of my own definition of who I am. It is an existential challenge. Being part of a medical group, a strategy ostensibly designed to survive the maelstrom of managed care, has transformed me from being an individual doctor, a physician who could rely on his own abilities and reputation, to being part of an amorphous whole, whose definition in the aggregate reflected the lowest common denominator of the group. In fact, I was now referred to as a provider, not a doctor, not a physician, but a provider. But, a provider of what? In my case it had little to do with healing; what we're talking about here is the provision of an health care event, one defined by a major dose of cost control, one defined by seeing a requisite number of patients per day, one defined by activating a system that promised to rush the patient off to some other specialty provider, or some other machine, which would inevitably serve as a poor substitute for a careful history and physical exam and which would ultimately substitute silicone chips, fiberoptics, and x-rays for a meaningful human encounter. I felt lost, submerged by the larger organization, defined by that group, a definition that I neither sought nor asked for, and that definition was the one patients referenced when we first met.

In 1996 I was a member of a hospital based HMO in Sacramento. I was asked to see a 31 year old man ostensibly for a second opinion regarding treatment options for intractable gastroesophageal reflux disease. This is situation where the lower esophageal sphincter is incompetent allowing an acid refluxate into the esophagus causing heart burn and occasionally marked inflammation, ulcers and cancer. The patient had been seen earlier by my gastrointestinal colleague in the downtown Sacramento office. The diagnosis was straight forward and the endoscopic findings were confirmatory, including macroscopic evidence of mucosal inflammation. His history was one of lifelong upper abdominal pain. This symptom had led to a previous gallbladder operation and cardiac consultations. The patient was appropriately treated by my colleague using antisecretory medication. A followup endoscopic study by me revealed complete healing. But the patent's pain persisted, which was the reason for the second opinion. He underwent further diagnostic studies that confirmed the diagnosis of GERD. The general surgeons in the downtown office did not believe that he was a surgical candidate, in part because of his endoscopic response to treatment and in part because of his atypical life long pain. I agreed with their reasoning and I felt that there was likely a psychological component to the pain. The patient thought otherwise and wanted surgery. By the time he saw me he was fed up with our group, feeling discounted and not receiving proper care. His take of our managed care group was less than flattering and he demanded to be seen by a surgeon outside of our group. I took this as a personal affront. Outsourcing is always frowned upon by managed care groups because it is not cost effective. We HMO doctors were salaried, which would not be the case with the outside surgeon who was bound to charge more should our group choose to underwrite the surgery. He actually did have the surgery done at his own expense. Unfortunately, he sustained a perforation during the procedure, but it was repaired and I was told that he ultimately did well. The point of all this is that this patient, like others I have seen, had a negative attitude regarding our HMO, which included all of the doctors he had seen. Being part of this HMO made me a part of the whole, not James Hansen, and thus a recipient of contempt before investigation.

The admonition to manage my time efficiently had been an ominous warning that the system's survival would eventually be triaged at the expense of any experience between the patient and physician; that the "good doctor" understood this and was invited to find ways to enhance efficiency, to eliminate wasteful interpersonal exchanges, to invent and learn how to operate machines that cut through the extraneous and get down to the Cartesian meat the matter. Horseface would have loved this.

Many of my new colleagues in this new managed care group practice venture were incompletely trained. Their general fund of knowledge was suspect. Managed care has given rise to physician organizations that simply need warm bodies, not necessarily competent physicians, warm bodies needed to fill the ranks of the primary care physician, those gate-keepers who stand between patients and specialists in an effort to control costs, but who actually stand to increase costs to the physician group when timely referrals are not made. This influx of young, compliant, naïve physicians is a cause for concern. Mediocrity has raised its ugly head, the antithesis of quality, where care is simply substituting a glitzy test or procedure for careful listening and empathy. As I have already discussed, during the past twenty years of teaching experience at UC Davis I noticed a subtle change in the focus or vision of new doctors. To tell you the truth, they seem less prepared. Or, put another way, they have a different set of skills. Computer literacy, net-working, and knowing how to get patients on the high tech juggernaut, rate high on their list.

Traditional basic science, a firm grasp of pathophysiology, pharmaceutical sophistication, and applied therapy seem shortchanged. There is a heavy dose of cynicism. The thought that anything short of high technology might serve the patient is discounted. This is an attitude fostered and nourished by the medical school faculty, as their own success is predicated on publishing articles about high technology as well as grinding out lucrative procedures. The real damage done is found within the makeup of the new physician. These new primary care physicians are less willing and able to make decisions on their own; they are incomplete doctors unless bonded to specialists, often technophysicians, with ready access to high technology; they readily assume a subservient role in the eyes of the patient, unable to offer authenticity, resolve, ingenuity, and caring.

The art form of medicine, the portion that included matters of the mind, the spiritual dimension, is conspicuously missing. Healing medicine is what took place between Dr. Fontaine and Mary Little. There was mutual respect, an invitation for a meaningful dialogue, a careful assessment, and a treatment plan that did not rush Mary Little off to high technology. There was patient contact; Dr.Fontaine touched Mary Little and looked into her eyes. He redefined his and her status to two concerned human beings, one of which was blessed with the skill and information needed to deal with the renal failure and the stroke and, at the same time, to redirect Mary Little towards a meaningful divine-human relationship.

During the years that I participated in the clinical outpatient gastroenterology service at UC Davis, there was a noticeable attitudinal change in resident behavior. Towards the end, when a resident was invited to critically evaluate a patient's complaint, there was a rush to get a note on the chart, to accept whatever I said without question, to prescribe whatever medicine I thought was appropriate, and to either admonish or patronize the poor patient who was usually bewildered, often unable to speak English, and not invited to communicate. I believe that some of this went on when I was a house officer, but this behavior seemed to become more prevalent during the years that I was involved in teaching. The evidence is strengthened by the attitude of physicians whose training has occurred during the past 25 years. There is a rush to judgment, a reach for high technology before engaging any spiritual strengths or at least trying out less invasive technology.

Managed care has had a discernable effect on the patient population seen in county hospitals. As we noted above, charitable care has been one of the underpinnings of professionalism. Access to care has generally been available to patients without means in large county hospitals, which have traditionally been the beneficiary of philanthropic dollars. Managed care, along with MediCare and MediCaid, has eclipsed this relationship; a relationship defined by free care to the patient where the quid pro quo was a willingness of the patient to be part of the teaching experience. Costs have risen so high, and remuneration has fallen so low, that charity hospitals have fallen on hard times. Patients who do manage to access teaching hospitals seem to intuitively know that they are often seen as a burden to both administrators and house officers. These under-served patients have always been heroes to my way of thinking. Although they were mostly unsophisticated, often at the bottom of the nation's food chain, and not infrequently unable to speak English, I always felt that they had an intuitive intelligence about what was going on. During all of the years that I was in training at Los Angeles County General Hospital, I never head any patient complain about being a 'guinea pig." It certainly doesn't take a fluency with English to make these complaints known. Sure, they didn't like being crowded together in halls or large wards; they didn't like the lack of privacy, the noise, and the lack of amenities. But, they were an active part of the doctor/patient relationship, readily compliant, willing to submit to our ministrations because of an indefinable faith, and a source of strength to those of us struggling to learn and help them at the same time. At the same time they were not afraid to ask questions about the direction of their health care, but the shear magnitude of the suffering, the huge number of patients, the scarcity of translators and the inevitable time constraints, all made meaningful communication a challenge.

There has also been an influx of offshore medical graduates who grab up the nearly 8000 extra residency slots every year. These are residency slots that are over represented by the gimmicks and gadgets of specialty medicine. The admonition to find a gimmick as a means to success has found a wider audience. There has been an immediate symbiosis between these aggressive proceduralists and timid primary care physicians, a relationship conveniently woven within the tapestry of managed care groups. These doctors fit in nicely with a large group practice. As physicians gather together, as they attempt to fend off the managed care savages circling their wagons, some doctors seem to thrive in a group, or at least survive, living well on rations, not venturing out beyond the fortifications, expert in defensive strategy. They work within the constraints of cost control, making decisions that are driven by the general group's attempt to hold down out of group referrals, secure in the knowledge that they are the only ones left to do the job. This new relationship, born of managed care, has substituted convenience for economic gain, which although itself a point of concern, had previously driven the engine of referral. In neither case has quality been well served. Managed care has created an opportunity for less than stellar physicians, who subtly blend in with the group, redefining the nature of the group, substituting mediocrity for authenticity, creating a new health care reality which not only confuses, but aggravates the patient, substituting a less palatable brand of medicine for the traditional fee-for-service model. Managed care has methodically and inexorably invaded the American health care universe. It appears that managed care will play a major role in the Obama health care plan where accountable care organizations will be the methodology.

Today's environment is ruled by prepayment even more than it was a mere five years ago. Physicians are placed at risk by the payers, and find themselves having to make decisions that are fiscally prudent, not necessarily sound, simply to survive. There is far less freedom. Although politicians talk about various governmental insurance schemes ostensibly leading to universal health care, governmental intervention never stops at the water's edge. These are simply a portal for more and more incursion and control.

The very notion of managed care rankles the sensibilities of many caring physicians; the supposition that lay individuals are capable of participating in the health care drama is anathema. My view is that physicians that see the practice of medicine as a job, rather than a vocation, are more comfortable with managed care, where cookbook medicine simplifies the situation. That concept simply didn't exist when I took my first steps into the foray of becoming a doctor. That I would share this sacred vocation with some business type, someone displaced from the scene, someone charged with controlling costs, and in so doing, sharing the physician's pen, was never a thought. Still, sharing the physicians pen with the patient does make sense, however. When Dr. Fontaine revealed the power and sanctity of problem solving for Mary Little, there was never a hint that lay individuals might some day play a role. Those physicians with whom I trained believed that we were the captain of the ship, and if the buck stopped anywhere, it was with them. Physician pride, which at times reaches the level of pomposity, has taken it in the shorts with managed care. Written orders, that most sacred element, are now summarily changed by some amorphous entity living on the dark side, some ill-defined creature lying deep within the lattice work of the HMO. Naturally, HMOs are smart enough to enlist the aid of physicians, not necessarily current and up-to-date, not necessarily familiar with the nuances of any particular specialty, rather mercenaries, who find it easier to sit in the shadows, inaccessible, and prostitute their signature for these outrageous and egregious decisions.

Take the case of Marge McGuire. She was a 58-year-old grandmother who was diagnosed by me as having gastroesophageal reflux disease. We have already discussed that this is where acid refluxes into the esophagus causing damage. Marge was given a prescription of Prilosec, 20mg to be taken daily, just before breakfast. She had immediate relief and was very grateful. However, several months later she called to say that the drug was no longer helping. I spent some time trying to understand why this was so. Sometimes it is because of compliance issues, weight gain, or other medications given by other physicians. Or, perhaps her symptoms are due to a new problem. Almost as an afterthought she related that her HMO had dropped her dose down to 10mg without telling anyone. This was heavy handed cost control by the payer who subtly misled the patient into believing it was my decision. I was furious. I tried not to betray my misgivings, but I could hardly put a complete sentence together. It was clear to me that her HMO was practicing medicine without a license. But, wait a minute. I'm sure that this directive was undersigned by one of those rent-a-docs. I eventually got her back on the right dose, but not without a fair amount of time and effort. I felt helpless, discounted, irrelevant, but mostly angry. This type of thing happens many times each day. Sometimes tests are denied, sometimes treatments are denied. HMOs have no reluctance to assault the doctor-patient relationship. Their financial success, their bottom line, is the issue, which emerges from an amoral cauldron, which may soon be controlled by government.

Physicians who are newly trained, like those I taught at UC Davis, often take much of this for granted. They have gone through their training left with a watered down concept of the doctor-patient relationship. Yet, in spite of the above, there were a number of seasoned physicians who were members of my group. Preauthorization is one of the draconian measures instituted to hold costs down. Since I am a specialist, I am asked to approve requests for CT scans, amongst other things, to approve of tests thoughtfully considered by my more experienced physician partners, a down right disgusting task given the fact that many of these doctors are more expert in ordering the damn things than myself. Sure, there are the marginal physicians referenced above, but, once again, managed care has dropped the ceiling for everyone. My mother was a grammar school teacher and she often complained about the frustration of adjusting the pace of teaching to the slowest learner. Maybe this is important to do in public education, but in a physician group, lowering expectations is one more cause for concern. Managed care attenuates the challenges that help physicians grow. There is no invitation to spend meaningful time with difficult cases, cases where the road marks are less clear, cases where groups of physicians meet in conference to share their experience and knowledge. Time management has replaced intellectual curiosity. Patients with complicated problems are either sent off to a specialist many times not in the group, passed off to the medical school, or hospitalized out of frustration.

We must drill deeper into the concept of managed care, to take a closer look at the *care* moiety. I spent several years on a steering committee created to facilitate a redesign of our hospital. We borrowed some of the techniques used in re-engineering corporations. Clinical guidelines or pathways were identified as measures suitable for physicians to work on and hopefully improve the organization's bottom line in a hostile economic environment. Given that value is a function of quality divided by cost, the charge to physicians was to massage this equation and increase value. We physicians, like others across the country, found within the methodology of Continuous Quality Improvement, a way to attack this problem. We learned that committees of doctors, sharing their thoughts and experience, could identify essential steps, which lay between the presentation of a patient with certain signs and symptoms, and the successful treatment of the disorder. This sequence of events was closely scrutinized in an effort to identify the most efficient processes hoping to reduce variation between providers, to improve quality, and to control costs. Errors were seen as systemic problems. The expectation was that science would validate each step in the process leading to best outcomes. These guidelines were thought to be most applicable to the least complex, most frequently seen and the most costly illnesses. This is still promulgated as the way to improve health care across America, but there is more to it than that.

Never mind that health care expenditures have not fallen during the past several years under managed care, never mind that the insurance industry is now trying to control the cost of health care by passing more of the risk to patients in the form of co-payments. The constraints of managed care leave little room for healing, for including the spiritual dimension. There is very little room for hope. Healing is more than aiming Ehrlich's magic bullet at the affliction, more than interrupting the cellular and subcellular events in the pathophysiologic scenario, more than correcting abnormal laboratory values. Healing is a global event, with a spiritual dimension, not impersonal, not occurring independent of the mind, and not necessarily measured by how well we can turn the clock back, as if the illness had never occurred. Healing is cost effective. Physicians who understand this are better stewards, do not simply rely on high technology, and make use of empathy, intuition, altruism and hope. Human Beings are substantially changed or different after any illness, no matter how great or small it is. Life is a process, modified by various vicissitudes, exigencies, challenges, successes, and failures. It is not static, nor should it be; the goal from the physician's point of view is to allow the body to heal, applying good science and including those strengths inherent in healing, and by alleviating suffering while all of this is happening. When appropriate, the full array of scientifically proven disease fighting techniques should be applied in concert with the elements of healing. Saving a life may not be the primary goal if the situation is futile, but healing efforts, which include hope, are always appropriate. However, we physicians have allowed the polluted winds of change to create this managed care monster. As important, we patients have allowed these winds of change to play havoc with our heath care system.

To be fair, there is some evidence that health indices improve with universal health insurance. There is also evidence that disparities among different ethnic and socioeconomic groups are lessened with universal health care. Blood pressure, blood sugar, serum cholesterol, even response to cancer treatment are some markers that have been studied and do improve. These are limited and do not come close to meaningful health, improved quality of life, and the battle with chronic disease. The costs born to government to achieve these improvements, albeit simplistic health care markers, will be exorbitant. I see the heavy hand of government subsidizing physician extenders and marginalizing meaningful holistic health care, care that borrows from the scientific method and is leavened with spirituality. The incentives for becoming a physician would be lessened and physician quality would be adversely affected. There will always be a need for highly trained physicians, those who use high technology appropriately, those who sustain the quality of life, in spite of aging and the inevitable burden of death. These physicians will become scarce. I believe in universal health care, but done by concerned physicians, physicians who are good stewards, who add a spiritual dimension to the practice of medicine, and in so doing, share this available power with their patients. Government has a constitutional obligation to insure the public welfare and to that extent has some duty to oversee the process, but not directly participate in it , assuming for itself the role of physician.

We have allowed health care engineers to define what is best for us, which is often what is best for the control costs at the expense of quality, and what seems attractive to the constituents of politicians whose major motivation is to get reelected. The time is now for we the people to stand up and be counted.

Chapter 14
Empathy—The Missing Ingredient

Meaningful rapport with suffering patients flows from genuine empathy, where much of the suffering inherent in chronic disease is alleviated, where an inordinate amount of health care dollars is spent with high technology that is not needed. There are many physicians who have neither possessed nor cultivated this tool. So many of us are wounded healers, unable to genuinely respond to our patient's misery, substituting a boiler plate rejoinder born from the need to protect our own inadequacies. The innate or spiritual gift of empathy may not be available; perhaps because of an impermeable and intransigent ego; perhaps because the struggles of the medical education process have tarnished this precious gift; or, alas, a conscious decision is made to subordinate this divine aspect of our being for reasons having to do with personal agendas or cost control.

One consequence of this sad state of affairs is the unadulterated misuse of high technology. Beneath the surface, quietly tucked away in the subconscious, is the specious and absurd assumption that the fortunes of medical advancement are able to replace the intuitive. In an instant the intimate and personal legacy of medicine is cast away. Yet, there are opportunities to recover and develop empathy, albeit limited, especially with busy practices where time is an important determinant of the bottom line and success or failure is predicated on cost control. Self-discovery is one first step along the journey towards the rediscovery or acquisition of empathy. Self-discovery is available in some way, in some time or place, to anyone who chooses to practice medicine. It may take some reflection. In my own case the process began with an early morning jog.

It would be my last run, obviously unknown to me when I began, an unwelcome realization, which was thankfully unavailable at the time, one that would crystallize soon enough. The cool morning air had not yet given way to the sun's rays, which promised another hot day. It was so much better to start before the sun climbed too high in the sky. These moments of solitude connected with a primordial part of my being and, for those instances, a release from life's meaner side, a vague promise of immortality. The run began as an extraordinary high, a temporary release from the onerous aspects of life, anticipating a delicious menu of thought. The rivulets of cool air anointed my skin, ever so gently, a respite from the heat of yesterday's blazing sun rising off the pavement. It was a sensory feast.

It was Easter morning, an appropriate time to reflect upon the gifts of renewal and rebirth. The fluidity of a runner's motion attests to God's creativity. Bipedal locomotion for homo sapiens, a product of our evolution, is a marvelous gift considering the awkward construction of our bodies. Our vertebral bodies sit precariously atop one another, a unique burden, given the force of gravity. Yet, it works, and with training, running is nearly effortless. The first half of the run was a joy. The shadows cast by the early sun felt like an intimate encounter with the power of the universe. A kinship between running and rebirth was revealed, as if the residue and baggage of yesterday was shed uncovering and revealing an essential newness.

The last five miles of the run, however, presented a new challenge. Like any runner I have had my share of aches and pains, reminders of mortality, and part of the process. On this occasion, however, the discomfort of the moment did not seem related to fatigue; it was a peculiar pain that intermittently involved my left leg. Stride and motor strength were intact. Yet, as I kept running there were more frequent sharp pains, which radiated down my left leg. The last mile or so became extremely tedious because of this discomfort, distorting an otherwise delicious moment, distracting and refocusing my thought process away from the cosmos and towards this limb. I eventually finished but with some difficulty.

I had two previous back surgeries because of sciatica and a herniated disc in the L4/L5 interface, the most recent having been several years previously. Accordingly, the nature of this pain in my left leg certainly caught my attention. Was this a recurrence of degenerative lumbar disk disease? Was this a new nerve root irritation? These were unsettling thoughts that broke through the usual revelry at the end of a run. For several days I dismissed the notion that there was a problem. Life merrily made its way along its well-traveled path while I ignored this five hundred pound gorilla sitting in the corner of my existence. Exercise done regularly and conscientiously leads to positive addiction, a paradoxically healthy habit, and often a temporary slide into withdrawal when it is denied. Much has been written about positive addiction; I might never have felt the pang of withdrawal without this little leg problem. The prudent choice was to temporarily stop running and develop some other low impact aerobic experience. Being such a creature of habit I found that hard to do. However, after trying to run on several subsequent occasions I finally got the message and gave it up. The neighborhood gym promised a plethora of aerobic equipment and was to be my new home.

The gym, filled with people of various shapes and sizes, wearing costumes ranging from boring to outlandish, bathed in loud pulsating music providing the background for the various grunts and groans, replaced the out-of-doors, the smell of flora, and the feeling of being one with the natural state of things. The cardiovascular stress required for conditioning is a function of sustained effort. Whether climbing a mountain, playing basketball, surfing, or whatever, the heart is indifferent, progressively more efficient with the force of contraction in meeting the increased metabolic needs of the body. People-watching replaced meditation, televisions replaced nature's vista, rock music replaced the chirp of birds, but the physiology remained constant.

Leg pain became a constant companion during the next several years. Initially, there was very little difficulty in walking or going to the gym. Swimming eventually replaced running, quietly and unobtrusively, without a whimper, without my realizing it, with no major protest from me. On a subconscious level the pain invited me to redraw the boundary lines of my life. Suddenly I no longer missed running, and in fact it was no big thing. Its central position was displaced by other physical activities, which were less painful. At the same time, right before my eyes, I had given up one of the greatest pleasures that I had. Here, now for me to see, was incontrovertible evidence of the innate ability of our species to adjust to chronic adversity when measured in physical pain. When survival of the species was paramount, adjusting to pain was essential. Athletes play hurt, competing effectively on the highest level while displacing their physical anguish to a lower level of consciousness. However, when the signs and symptoms of disease are ignored, an attitude more characteristic of men than women, it is a guarantee of worse to come.

Personally, I always felt that there was an invisible shield around my own body, which would protect me from adversity and provide me with immortality. There was always a safe distance between Matilda and myself. I was at least conceptually aware of the possibility of illness and death but these thoughts were abstract in nature, which I infrequently but occasionally mulled over in my mind. When one of my patients suffered a bad outcome, the trilogy of death, disability and disease reached out in a sinister and malevolent fashion, but the invidious invader could not penetrate my denial, which was so tenaciously protected. The pain in my left leg did not actuate any creative or introspective thought; it was a nuisance, meaningless, unconnected to my concept of myself.

For the next several years I made subtle adjustments in my work environment. I began to sit for most of my procedures and to walk more slowly. There was no perceptible limp or, at least I was unaware of one, so the secret was mine. But the secret was so buried in my subconscious that it was essentially hidden from me. I had become one of those human beings who unknowingly reorganize their lives to accommodate a physical disability. As a physician I have seen patients make amazing adjustments, made without an overt decision, designed to palliate physical disabilities without requiring the sufferer to jump out of the stream of life. Patients with swallowing disorders subtly change the consistency of their food, subsisting on pureed preparations for many years, without being consciously aware of it. Others with visual and auditory disorders somehow make adjustments in their life that subordinates these disabilities to a fundamental need to carry on. I am reminded of a patient with chronic diarrhea, whose life was punctuated by multiple calls to evacuate, whose job as a postman required him to have memorized every toilet along his route, the distance between each, how much time each stop would take, and yet, he rarely gave this predicament a second thought.

My office in Sacramento was approximately two hundred yards from the hospital and the endoscopic suite. I began each day with several endoscopic procedures. On this particular morning, a gray, dismal, and cold day, I began my walk from the parking structure adjacent to the building, which houses my office, to the hospital. My mornings are routine and have been for a number of years, but I was very aware that I was conspicuously late. This fact was not lost on the family of my first patient who admonished me for my tardiness. Accosted by a very unhappy wife, as I made my way to the endoscopic suite, intent in knowing where I had been, she stepped into the adjoining hallway, still bundled up in her winter clothes, a face devoid of softness, a mixture of apprehension and anger, and said,

"Dr. Hansen, my husband was here one hour prior to the procedure, as your office insisted, and that was ninety minutes ago. We are both very nervous and upset."

For such a diminutive woman she was the antithesis of diffidence. Her eyes focused upon mine, she stood her ground, not willing to surrender the moment or space, carefully awaiting my reply. I was taken aback. There was no real reason for my tardiness except that I was now walking more slowly for reasons which were becoming far more clear to me. My recollection of this encounter has left me with the distinct impression that, besieged by this woman, my pain was now more noticeable. During the interval wherein I gathered my wits, not wanting to be flip or disingenuous in my response, my mind's eye recalled walking more slowly because of the pain. My insipid response was "I'm sorry. I have a pain in my left leg, which makes walking more tedious and I am afraid that I walk a bit more slowly".

In this instance the truth seemed to assuage her. This was clearly an epiphany for me. There was no getting around the fact that I had a physical disability. All of my defense mechanisms and attempts to bury information into my subconscious were laid bare and crying for recognition. These thoughts were competing for the attention demanded by the procedure, which happily was completed without difficulty and with a good outcome. The patient and his wife were elated, all vestiges of unhappiness swept away, but the residue of uncertainty was left for me. What should I do? I needed help.

I returned to the neurosurgeon who had done my first two lumbar laminectomies and who was a friend. His examination was somewhat cursory, but at least he did something—he ordered an MRI of my lower back. He didn't exactly examine me, he actually didn't listen much to me or make meaningful eye-contact, but he did something. That proved to be a frightening experience. Claustrophobia complicated the experience; the narrow confines of the menacing machine reduced any pretense of clarity to a non-nondescript, amorphous primordial fear, albeit ill defined, but nonetheless operative. This procedure led me to the other side of the divide that exists between the doctor and patient. This was a difficult transformation for me. The insight and information, which I possessed about a wide range of medical conditions, was made useless, irrelevant, a learning that was neither prescient nor sagacious, only experiential. My musing during that procedure led me to the concept of surrender, a release of control, a requirement, but anathema to physicians. I was being asked to submit to this test, or any other, knowing full well the range of possible complications. No longer an abstract concept, my task demanded that I let go of my need to call the shots. Miraculously, I survived. But I was alone, the only help came from the technician who played soft music during the procedure.

Back in my neurosurgeon's office we reviewed the MRI, as if I could understand all of the subtle shadows, and I asked,

"Tony, so what's the verdict?"

He took the time to show me the results of my previous surgeries–– marked scoliosis of my spine, the wreckage of my arthritis and the treatments, excessive calcification and narrowing of the foramina through which coursed the lumbar and sacral nerve roots.

"Jim, it's not good but I believe that there is something that we can do about this.'

"Jesus, what is that supposed to mean, I thought? Something like cut the leg off?"

There was a distinct vacuum in our dialogue. After what seemed an interminable interval, Tony went on to tell me that a third neurosurgical procedure in this area would be more difficult, more hazardous, and with a less secure prognosis, but possible. Again my brain exploded, "possible, like surviving a shark attack?" It was a bit unsettling, to say the least. I recalled other physicians admonishing potential back patients to consider the services of a psychiatrist before submitting to a third back operation. This bit of cynicism encodes some truth. His plan was to release one or other nerve roots from their stenotic foramina and thereby eliminate my pain. With mixed emotions, like every patient, I wanted the reassurance that the procedure was fail–safe, an unrealistic expectation, and that the outcome would be secure. Naturally, he couldn't give me that reassurance. Tony and I danced around the uncertainty of surgery, with neither spiritual nor emotional contact between us, allowing the decision–making process to play out on a more superficial level, finding refuge from the immediacy of the moment in non–decision. This non-decision robbed me of the process of becoming, making those subtle changes in attitude that would augment healing. In my experience, patients who are short changed like this have a more difficult time with postoperative healing and with adjusting to the functional changes wrought by surgery. Not relishing the thought of surgery, this approach had some appeal. Upon leaving his office I felt empty and crest–fallen. My interpretation of what he said was that he was committing me to a life of pain and disability. This was hard to swallow. Could I be barking up the wrong tree? Was Tony unsure of himself? Was his conservative approach a way out of his own insecurity?

There was no essential bond between the two of us. It was if we were communicating by Morse Code. The words were intelligible and comprehensible, but without meaningful connection. Tony's body language was anything but soft and inviting. The eddy currents of air that circulated between and around us were cold and uncomfortable. He might as well have delivered his assessment with a megaphone high on a cliff. His smile was perfunctory; it seemed contrived and difficult to hold in place. This unsettling detente forced me to fold the edges of this experience and tuck them away. Being the patient changed my focus from problem solving to being compliant. I certainly did not want to create angst in my doctor, the person who might be the one that operated on me. By the same token, I did not want to adulterate his decision making process. I certainly had an advantage being a physician, an advantage that allowed me to closely follow his thinking, but like all patients I needed to feel comfortable with the process and invited to be a part of the process.

Now the pain began the journey from my subconscious to my conscious mind; it claimed a greater measure of my resources. It was most apparent when walking or changing positions; sitting continued to provide respite. I was taking increasing amounts of non–steroidal anti-inflammatory agents, which led to the predictable side effects of tinnitus and diaphoresis. The subtle and malicious nature of the pain and its inexorable march into my consciousness eventually demanded a call to arms. What was I waiting for? My attitude became a hostage to the pain. A number of patient complaints were brought to my attention: poor communication; poor attitude; unresponsive. When asked to see another patient in consultation, I mostly whined and tried to wiggle out of it. I was now nearly totally consumed by this invidious affliction. How could I continue to practice medicine? What would I do with my life? These morbid preoccupations germinated, leaving pernicious buds to spread the pollen of discontent. I vacillated between self–flagellation and self- pity. I found myself totally at the mercy of this illness.

The opportunity to discover the meaning of my situation fell to assuaging my pitiful circumstance. An opportunity to shift my focus from the purely physical aspects of the problem to the discovery of potential emotional or spiritual causes became a casualty. Driven by the fear of obsolescence or non-relevancy, I fantasized an ignominious end to my career. A prisoner of my training, thoroughly indoctrinated in the nuances of western medicine, the succor of conventional allopathic medicine eclipsed potential alternative options. This prejudice foreclosed other approaches, which may have fed me spiritually, provided me with additional insight, and helped me choose a more intrepid and salubrious path. My physician was of no help in these matters. I had the same feelings when confronted by Horse Face so many years ago. Judy Springer invited empathy. I do remember the feelings, but so vague, so long ago.

During my reign as chief-of-staff, which had occurred several years previously, I had the unenviable task of brokering a peace between the neurosurgeons and a brash, young back surgeon named Bruno Piazza. The issue was whether or not to grant certain privileges regarding specialized surgical procedures on the axial spine to Dr. Piazza. These included fairly sophisticated anterior and posterior plating procedures to stabilize areas of the spine in persons with various congenital, arthritic, or traumatic conditions. These were the type of operations, when done in a cavalier way that led to the downfall of Dr. Nigel Southworth. These procedures had heretofore been the exclusive province of neurosurgeons who were not necessarily up to date and proficient in the more recent modifications, but who claimed the privilege by birth-right. This was clearly a political issue, a turf issue, and one that had strong overtures of economics. Piazza, however, was highly trained. He had been on the faculty at the medical school where he had authored a number of important papers and had been involved with teaching the nuances of these procedures to senior residents. He had also been involved in the research and development of several of the advanced techniques. He was cocky, smug, insolent, and definitely not a team player. The neurosurgeons insisted that one must be a neurosurgeon, a member of their club, to be granted these privileges. Of course, Piazza had a different point of view since he was fundamentally an orthopedic surgeon; and he firmly staked his claim. Initially, a very tenuous compromise was reached and each side tired of the argument. Soon thereafter Piazza won out because no one on the other side felt compelled to carry on.

Wrestling with the recommendations I had received for my own problem, I decided to seek a second opinion. Piazza was the man. He was gracious enough to see me on rather short notice, one of the egregious perks of being a colleague, a consultation ordained by my previous stature as chief-of-staff. He immediately had new x-rays taken of my lower spine spending most of the session examining these as well as my MRI. The initial conversation was limited, punctuated by small talk, interspersed with Piazza engaging himself in conversation. He was short and fat, with ill-fitting clothes, appearing uneasy and in constant motion. He shifted from one foot to the other, humming while studying the radiographs, looking terribly important, infused with an abundance of self-confidence, but with very little eye contact. Suddenly, he blurted,

"Jim, this is not a good back.

As if I didn't know it. Once again taking a private tour of my back, he mumbled,

"This will take two surgeries."

I didn't need to hear that. I cannot recall the rest of the conversation. Two operations, two separate opportunities for inadvertent complications, two major surgical procedures on a decimated lumbar spine. He was nevertheless reluctant to take the first step, to embark upon these procedures, to advise anything. In one sense it was another reprieve, a chance to mull over the proposal; I was relieved, yet, dissatisfied.

Where would I go now? What would I do now? Two highly respected physicians agreed that there was a chance for improvement with surgery, but there was reluctance. These guys usually operated in a second, rushing headlong into the technological fray, never looking back. But, in my case, there was a sense of inertia.

I did not feel part of the solution. As a patient, even as a somewhat informed patient, I was not invited to participate in the decision making process. I believe that all patients need to be invited to participate in their own health care. This invitation not only provides solace, but it insures compliance. It was like being left out in the cold while others deliberated my fate. There was an overwhelming feeling of powerlessness.

Now totally consumed with pain, less mindful of those who needed my help, my days were spent adjusting to this reality. It was no longer a subconscious experience. I had crossed another threshold. The vagaries of life have very little patience for individuals with chronic pain. This new experience became a personal test tube inviting me to find a way out. Alchemy replaced reason. How could I transform the pain into some other less onerous experience? This presupposed that I had a modicum of control over the situation and that a willful decision would be efficacious. I set sail to adjust my own microenvironment. The difficulty was in balancing the energy required to pull this off with that needed to successfully practice medicine. I was caught in an unhappy dichotomy. I discovered that chronic pain feeds off of secondary gain. In my case there was a need to have external reassurance that I was indeed suffering. Alchemy served me well insofar as I could convert the response of those around me into pity.

My nurse periodically kept track of my discomfort.

"Dr. Hansen, have you taken your medicine today? You are limping more that usual. How do you manage? How can you keep going?"

My contrived response would be,

"Linda, it's no big thing. It seems to get better during the day. I don't think I need any medication."

All the while I was hoping that she wouldn't lose track of the seriousness of my situation.

It was high theater. Without a meaningful connection to any of my physicians, I was left to my own devices.

This dialogue was played out daily. Now, the dance of alchemy had center stage. I was willfully manipulating my environment to prop up the pity from without and thereby transform the pain into a new reality, which integrated the pain into my total being.

Totally unprepared for the outcome, I found myself in conversation with one of the hospital nurses with whom I worked and who had certainly heard me complain more than once. It was a quiet day, there were a number of empty beds in the ICU where she worked. She was writing in the charts of her patients to the background of the incessant monitoring machines, when she suddenly lifted up her head and had the audacity to speak out,

"Dr. Hansen, let me give you the name of a physician who works downtown and specializes in backs. Perhaps a new face and a new perspective would be worthwhile."

Here was a person stepping out of my carefully choreographed environment, daring to suggest a change, unwilling to confine herself to my manipulations. Why couldn't I think of this. Again, the transformation to being the patient makes it a right brain experience, rather than a left brain experience. In other words, everything that I knew from being a physician did little to sooth my soul, to put me at ease, and to provide me with answers. I was seeking a meaningful bond with my physician. At least, in my case, I did not need collegiality from my physician at that moment, rather support and empathy.

I answered, "So what makes you think this guy would be better than the ones that I have?"

She answered, "It seems like anyone would be better than the ones that you have seen."

That felt like a blow to the solar plexus. It took my wind away. Suddenly breathless, but attempting to regain control, I hadn't scripted her response--but there it was. I took the name of this physician and changed the subject. Had the pain now become more important than its relief? Was it now an integral part of my existence in such a way as to require its preservation? Does this inevitably happen with chronic pain? Is this what happens when physicians don't conscientiously deal with their patients? I wrestled with these questions for the next several weeks. They became my companions, my bedfellows; and the Harpies cried for a response. I discovered that when totally consumed with self pity, the receiver of a telephone becomes an extraordinarily heavy object to lift. To reach out and connect with other human beings was at best a frightening proposition notwithstanding the fact that meaningful communication posits solace for the anguished heart.

An appointment was made. There was a singular request for a bone scan, which was unsettling, yet a departure from the usual itinerary. A bone scan is a painless procedure, an imaging study wherein a radioactive agent, tagged to an inert substance, is injected into the body. Depending on the organ to be studied, the material localizes, and in this case, throughout my skeleton. The images display changes that mirror whatever abnormality may exist. This provides the clinician with added information regarding the nature of whatever disturbance may exist.

I had the exam performed at the hospital. Later that morning, a very busy morning, I was examining one of my patients in my office when Linda interrupted me and told me that the nuclear medicine physician was on the phone. In general, I disdained telephone interruptions while examining patients and it was doubly disturbing since there was nothing about this scan, which portended any significant change in my diagnosis--at least, in my mind. With trepidation I lifted that otherwise ponderous receiver and said,

"Hi, Dave. What's up?"

David Wright was a very knowledgeable nuclear medical physician whose credentials included board certification in both internal medicine and radiology. Being a delightful person, originally from Philadelphia, he shared my enthusiasm about baseball. He was a die-hard Phillies fan. On more than one occasion we debated the subject of whether or not Pete Rose should be admitted to the Hall Of Fame. Dave believed that his performance transcended any other issue and should determine the outcome. Thus, he was in favor of this proposition. I took the opposite position, namely, that the integrity of the game was predicated upon preserving ethical and moral ballast. Since Shoeless Joe Jackson was denied admission to the Hall, I believed that Rose should suffer the same fate. We agreed to disagree and that's the way things have stood over the years. But, this phone call had nothing to do with baseball, Pete Rose, or the Hall Of Fame.

"Jim, I want you to come over now to the department so I can get an x–ray of your hip."

I answered, "My *hip*. You mean just waltz out of my office with all of these patients?"

His steadied response was, "Yes, I'm concerned about this scan. It won't take long. Just make some adjustments in your office schedule and you'll be back to finish without difficulty."

That was easy enough for him to say. What choice did I have? All of the juices of my essential uncertainty were released. The echoes of temerity rattled through my head. My modus had always included the need to create catastrophe out of nothingness. I immediately came to the conclusion that I had inoperable cancer.

Without giving it another thought I made the necessary changes in my schedule and hobbled over to the x–ray department. At the same time I wondered if this was the time to go coffin shopping. One of the x–ray technicians was awaiting my arrival and within a short period of time I was in the x–ray suite. Several pictures of my hip were taken. I quickly got dressed and returned to the waiting room where I waited to talk to Dr. Wright. He brought in both the recent bone scan and hip x-ray. He explained the situation as he saw it. The bone scan revealed an area of increased uptake of the radioisotope in the area of the left hip, a hot spot, the area known as joint space for the acetabulum and the head of the femur. It suggested either advanced degenerative joint disease or avascular necrosis. That was what bothered him. Avascular necrosis would demand immediate attention to both hips. Avascular necrosis is a result of poor blood supply to the head of the femur because of narrowing of the feeding vessel. The reasons are often obscure, although alcoholism is certainly one association. That certainly caught my attention. However, a marked collapse of the head of the femur, characteristic of avascular necrosis, was not apparent on my films, and thus early surgical intervention was not indicated. Thank God! In my case the arthritis in my left hip had left the bones in the joint space denuded of the articular cartilage, which provides lubrication for joint motion. The x–rays revealed bone on bone. This was confusing and hard to fit in with my back problems. Baseball aside, I still felt alone. The next stop was to the new orthopedic surgeon recommended by the nurse.

This guy was pleasant enough, but an inscrutable Asian, without much levity, but very efficient. With refreshing expertise, a new explanation for my leg pain was proffered. Carefully assimilating the historical, physical, and laboratory facts, a plausible case was made for my hip being the main cause of my misery. Now I was beginning to feel stupid. I had bought the back theory hook, line, and sinker. I'm supposed to know and understand this stuff. Having made the transition to being a patient, I shared with all patients the trust we freely give our physicians. Now I felt broadsided. The road marks were gone. Without any reservation, a surgical procedure was recommended, not on my spine, but on my hip. Somewhat timidly I asked, "What type of surgical procedure?"

He measured his words carefully, giving thought to my naive question, and answered, "Nothing less that a total hip replacement would do."

My only thought was that I would forever be activating the metal detector machines in airports. I pondered the plight of my amputated bone––A burial? A cremation? An ignominious end in a dumpster? Would death be shortchanged by the premature removal of one of my body parts?

The orthopedic surgeon suggested another Asian; a soft-spoken and attentive specialist in hip surgery. He was very gentle, but the gentleness applied only to my bodily tissues. He delicately touched my hip and the surrounding structures with the finesse of a master craftsman, however he was adamant regarding the notion that the only answer was a hip replacement. At one point in our conversation I believe that a tear fell from my eye. I was petrified that he might notice it. I was now convinced that the real problem was the hip. I envisioned headlines in the morning paper, "HANSEN'S PROBLEM THE HIP, NOT THE BACK. " So, not only did I have to deal with issue of a wrong diagnosis, but I was facing having one of my body parts removed.

What satisfaction it would be to see the faces of all my other surgeons when they read the headlines. By now I was out of options, at least options that seemed reasonable. The facts seemed to indict my hip. I wrestled several days with the proposition of hip surgery, what it would mean to record hip replacement amongst my list of personal illnesses, whether there would forever be a grating noise when I walked, and whether I would list to one side. In retrospect, none of my musing made much sense. I was a fighter on the ropes, waiting to be saved by the bell. I gave in and consented to the hip surgery, wondering if this would be the biggest mistake in my life.

After the hip surgery it wasn't long before I revisited the scene of my last run. The bike trail was unchanged. In fact, the trees, bushes, rocks, and river were unchanged, unaware of my plight and travail. The vista was unchanged, oblivious to the events surrounding my hip. My misgivings and fear had not altered the rhythmic ebbs and flow of nature. This time I retraced that last run on my bicycle. I had been advised to give up running which was anticlimactic anyway. But the pain was gone. That much was different. And, this occurred without any essential bonding with any of my physicians. So, what was the big deal? Somewhere, deep down inside, I learned that the process of becoming, the process of inculcating a new reality, was as important as the end result. The warmth and inner peace that accompanies meaningful rapport with other human beings had been truncated. Yes, my pain was gone, but I had no reference for which to deal with this new reality, that part of my body had degenerated to the point that it needed to be discarded: That part of my physical being had been chipped away and replaced with a glaring, new notion of my mortality. I felt shortchanged. As I rode along, my life unfolded before my eyes, a retrospective review of multiple patient encounters, a stark realization in living color that meaningful communication was often absent with my own interactions. I was gripped by a profound sadness. How many of my patients had been shortchanged? Yet, the road ahead was unchanged, an invitation to grab hold of these learnings before time ran out, and celebrate the gift of empathy.

It took many years to unlearn the lessons I learned from Horse Face. Horse Face's admonitions were so integrated within the interstices of my being, that it took my hip, the surgery, and this entire process to undo what had been so firmly entrenched early in my career. This was an essential turning point in my life as a physician. There are no coincidences and it took this complicated event to open my eyes. The small flame that flickered ever so slightly within my soul during that initial encounter with Mary Little and Dr. Fontaine, germinated and helped me to sort out this essential problem with health care. In retrospect it was the unsolicited empathy of the ICU nurse that led me to the proper course of action. She listened and connected with me. She taught me that empathy is the servant of science, adding to both the analytical and emotional aspects of healing. This led me to the understanding that empathy is one of the missing elements with modern allopathic medicine.

I now had a rudimentary foundation to support the rest of my journey, to make the case that our health care problems originate at this point of service. President Obama wants to fix the health care debacle, an admirable goal, but the perturbation originates at this point of service, and this is the place to focus. The next chapters continue the journey.

Chapter 15
The Wounded Healer: Reaching Beyond

Something gets lost during the arduous process of becoming a physician; incomplete personalities and moral asymmetry are the residue that provides a glimpse of what may be the lowest common denominator in the search for the cause of the health care crisis. Medical student's lives are so wrapped up in the process of mastering reductionist methodology that holism and common sense become casualties. Striving to understand and interpret pathophysiology, to understand the cellular and subcellular basis of disease, distorts the notion of healing. Balance becomes weaker, which leads to discomfort and reticence when confronted with the intangible aspects of humanness. The lust for a successful cure is a short-lived high eclipsing any hope of healing. Fundamentally, we physicians have lost contact with our souls. But, how does this happen? Alas, we ultimately become what we so diligently study, namely a mechanistic version of Homo sapiens, indifferent to metaphysics or any connection to a cosmic higher power, locked in a futile struggle to simply rewire broken circuitry. Healing includes genuinely caring for another human being. It includes the concept of shared suffering, the physician putting himself into the shoes of the patient, attempting to understand the pitfalls of illness. Physicians with a meaningful relationship with a higher power do not simply rely on high technology. Prayer and meditation provide the physician with power not otherwise available. Healing does not eliminate high technology, it downsizes it. It includes careful case selection, where the physician balances intrusive medicine with bedside medicine. Healing replaces many high technology procedures with simply listening, touching, smiling, eye contact, empathy and altruism. This is not so much an alternative approach as one that should always be included at the point of service, where doctor and patient meet. This is shared suffering. But, the educational process itself profoundly affects the new physician's attitudes and focus and the concept of shared suffering is left waiting at the gate. As a house officer, an intern and resident at Los Angeles County General Hospital, I learned how to deal with my patients very efficiently, managing my time carefully, heeding the advice given to me by Horseface, namely that matters of the mind are to be subordinated to culling out the malevolent invader.

As we became more proficient our tight tether was loosened. Some of our skills were extracted from Mother; others were a gift of grace. This learning process introduced us to the highs and lows of doctorhood. Wild vacillating swings of emotion accompanied efforts to cure patients. Healing was out of the question. These emotional swings follow us throughout our careers. However, we do not have meaningful emotional ballast to flatten out the peaks and valleys. I believe this robs us of serenity, joy, and fulfillment. A meaningful relationship with a higher power provides ballast.

A cardiac arrest case is illustrative. I'm not sure how I came upon him, what I was doing there, whether or not he was an assignment, but there he was, not breathing, blue, with no pulse. He was in this giant hospital, Los Angeles County General Hospital, on one of the wards, but we might as well have been two people on a deserted desert island. More than two sojourners in space, one of us was dying and the other, I, with an opportunity to save him. Aware of my surroundings and of the eyeballs fixed upon us, yet for a moment unable to transcend the inertia, which often accompanies fear, I made a deliberate and calculated move to his bedside. I was the only health care person around and if anything other than death was to supervene, I was the guy. Before I knew it I was deep into cardiopulmonary resuscitation. Here was this patient, about to cross over, being restrained by my nascent efforts.

Before long the area was a filled with urgency, equipment moving on wheels, the baleful cry of monitors looking for signs of life, and the PA system blaring "code blue." All of these technicians and nurses had been through this many times, but not me. For a moment I was unwilling to relegate my part of the CPR scenario to others because that would expose my thinking to all who were present. Mouth to mouth resuscitation actually gave me respite and a chance to search my brain for the next best thing to do. All of the tools were there: the defibrillator; medicines to stimulate or slow down the heart; endotracheal tubes to place in the trachea; a massive, complicated appearing breathing machine.

The EKG was the key. The fog dissipated enough for me to realize that the key was whether this was cardiac standstill, no electrical activity, or ventricular fibrillation, that rapid, uncoordinated, ineffectual pumping of the heart. In either event, his tissues were crying out for oxygen, for life-sustaining hemoglobin, the elixir of life. I stepped back.

The respiratory technician continued ventilation with a mask attached to a bag, which she compressed periodically delivering oxygen to the tissues. The EKG revealed ventricular fibrillation. I would need the paddles for defibrillation. I had never handled them but I knew that they generated electrical current, which needed to be passed through his chest and heart in an effort to restore a normal cardiac rhythm. What I knew at that time in my training came from watching my mentors or practicing on cadavers and dummies, where there was no life force at issue, Ventricular fibrillation occurs when the normal pacemaker system of the heart gives way to uncoordinated, non propulsive, contractions that originate in the ventricles.

I placed the paddles on his chest. We all stepped back aware of unwanted shocks possible with discharge. Now in full control, now sensing a leadership position, I barked, "discharge." Instantly, his body arched upward, an involuntary groan was audible, we all gasped. I was reminded of murderers being executed in the electric chair. But, this was a fleeting thought. Amazingly, the EKG revealed that his normal rhythm had been restored. He began to breathe spontaneously. For just a moment I believed that I had reordered the cosmos, placing myself on the celestial side of the divine-human encounter. I had saved a life, or at least I thought so, and now could start ascending Mt. Olympus. This was heady tonic, better than gin and tonic, and for a short period I was content. Until that moment the only human experiences which offered that much of a "high" were an orgasm, putting on after-ski boots, and a clean base hit, not necessarily in that order. Now, saving a life went to the top of the list. But, did I actually save a life?

The rub was that there were no congratulations, no parades, and no blaring headlines. I needed some sort of recognition. Resentment was slowly replacing the warm, intoxicating glow of success. Saving a life was not good enough, I needed more, some sort of pay off, an expectation was born in my mind and leaving a bitter taste in my mouth. Within a short period of time I was back to square one, somewhat more content than usual, but closer to neutral. This was a life-saving event, but something seemed to be missing.

A short moment later a senior cardiology resident arrived, the coronary care nurses took over the resuscitative effort, and Mr. X was whisked away to the CCU. He was still unconscious, but his vital signs were now normal, he was breathing on his own, and things looked good. Nobody paid much attention to me. I seemed to be in the way of the transportation team. Didn't these people know what I had done? Couldn't someone speak on my behalf? My supervising resident eventually arrived, quizzed me about what had taken place, nodded, and said "let's go", meaning it was time for rounds. That was it?

I was left with a vague feeling of unrest. What more did I need? Sure, it would have been gratifying for the Los Angeles Times to run a front page article about the event. But, there was something else. I have given this much thought over the years. What was absent was the healing aspect of this drama. If I had entered the fray bolstered by prayer I would surely have given thanks and the reciprocal feeling would have been a source of peace, joy and serenity. But I was unaware that prayer and meditation were important. Sure, the heart was restarted, and the patient survived. I am now convinced that a meaningful connection with a higher power, one nourished by prayer and meditation, is always appropriate, whether or not the patient is able to communicate. I have come to understand that there are a myriad of factors, which lead to heart disease, some which are amenable to allopathic medicine, but others which beg for metaphysical intervention: the power of hope, shared suffering, the strength inherent in empathy. In this case, maintaining a post resuscitation relationship would have been beneficial for both the patient and myself, but I made no effort and I had no information that it would have been helpful. I believe that we short-change our patients when we confine ourselves to standard reductionist intervention. And, why do we confine ourselves to reductionism? Because we have become what we have learned. Medical school curriculum is so weighted toward curing that there is no time or will to explore spiritualism, about healing efforts, and this most important relationship with a higher power. The years of intensive training have in some way rewired our own circuitry, leaving us out of contact with spiritual or metaphysical forces, which are available and cement the healing process. We have settled for a cure, starting the heart, and opted out of healing, the restoration of the whole organism. Here we begin to understand the nature of the wounded healer, the healer that practices medicine without any connection to a higher power, wounded because mastering reductionist methodology is seen as giving our best. It is not! There is something missing. We strive for bigger and better "saves"; we become votaries of high technology, which supplants the spiritual side of the equation. We don't talk to our patients, don't touch them, and don't cry with them. But the soulful physician does because he understands the nature of illness and he is connected to a higher power.

This case, like so many others, tug at the edges of that compensatory comfort zone new physicians try to create, assuring some semblance of sanity to what seems insane, and deftly covering over the blemishes which remain as a testament to the xenophobia of modern health care.

These emotional highs and lows seem to be an inevitable outgrowth of caring for other human beings. The trick for new doctors, physicians in training, is to dampen this emotional vacillation, which at times threatens objectivity. Over the years I have seen various ways physicians have buttressed themselves against these swings, or at least the lows. We learned different techniques during those formative years, which would last a lifetime. Without some type of cosmic purpose, spiritual identity, or some relationship to a higher power, the developing physician is easy prey for malevolent forces, which include greed, control, and self service, and which have the potential to change motive and focus and to barter emotional homeostasis for secular pragmatism; an effort to maintain balance in a sea of discord, a certain casualty of becoming what we study. We have learned how to become insulated and protected from otherwise healthy emotions. Some of this behavior has led to events that have profoundly changed health care, the role of the physician, and events, which portend future discontent.

I see very difficult cases. I am often stumped. Sometimes a referral to a tertiary center solves the problem. But, more often than not, meaningful answers are not there either. My life has changed a great deal since my training years. I am much more willing to seek out answers from my higher power, answers that are always there, if I am willing to ask. This presupposes that we doctors understand that we are not in complete control, that prayer and meditation are always appropriate, and that we would find that this higher power can do for us what we are not able to do ourselves. This is in essence aligning ourselves with God's will, which at best is an afterthought. This is anathema to today's physicians, and most especially the technophysicians. The notion has been bought and sold that science will ultimately provide answers leading to immortality.

This mindset is a subset of humanism, which posits that human beings will continue to improve as a species because of their inherent capacity to learn, that learning will lead to benevolence and serenity, and all we need to do is to provide the building blocks for the universal process of learning. Sadly, that has not been the case. Democracy, education, and a healthy environment, have not reduced wars, terrorism, illness, and man's quest for control. Maybe it will happen in time. My own experience is that spiritual solutions are readily available and infallible, but cast aside or ignored.

As a species, our DNA is not terribly different from a fruit fly. How is it then that we are so different physically, emotionally, and intellectually? Obviously, 600 million years of evolution have contributed significantly. Our brains are one of the most important phenotypic manifestations of our peculiar DNA. These brains are the substrate for the modifications that are acquired, or "nurture", which makes us so different. However, some of our uniqueness is attributable to spiritual forces which, like gravity, tugs at our souls seeking for a détente with the universal, that celestial power that seems so distant, yet a power that has clearly helped shape mankind. This gift provides us with the ability to transcend the physical, to establish a meaningful connection with higher power, to get answers, help and guidance from that higher power. Human beings appear to be the only species that has access to a spiritual dimension. We have a higher power with whom we can connect using prayer and meditation. This higher power requires faith, a peculiarly human asset, along with hope, meaning and inner peace. It is not synonymous with religion, although spiritualism can be found within religion. It is a connection with the cosmos, which is a requisite for healthy living. During the Age of Faith this was understood. Now, science is king, born of the enlightenment; humanism rules, rational thought and secularism holds sway, while spiritualism is relegated to the dump heap.

Part of the evolution of our species, as well as other species, is a "fight or flight mechanism." The hypothalamus is a part of the brain designed to sense danger. When danger is perceived hormones are released from the hypothalamus that activate the adrenal gland and the expression of cortisol and adrenergic hormones such as adrenaline. This is an autonomic response, it does not require involvement of the higher reaches of the brain, it simply senses danger and prepares us with heightened awareness and vigilance, clearer vision, and an increased pulse rate and blood pressure anticipating an encounter. This is a basic survival mechanism, but it is over stimulated in our complex environment. Instead of the fear of a wooly mammoth, our enemies are the stress of a unhappy partner, the ire of our boss, unpaid bills, unruly children, and the inevitable pain that accompanies age. Many of the chronic diseases, including chronic fatigue, irritable bowel syndrome, headache and insomnia are due to multiple "small emergencies" that activate the "flight of fight mechanism" and lead to constant stimulation by this system and its hormones. This constant stimulation drains our fuel tanks and ultimately perpetuates the problem. Technophysicians find this group of patients a tempting substrate for applying technomedicine, which is the basic problem.

The marvelous tools that we have at our disposal offer our species options for acting out in helpful and harmful ways. That is not the case with other animals and species whose instinctual behavior is survival-oriented. For instance, in Konrad Lorenz' book, *On Aggression*, we learn that intra-species battles rarely leave a dead loser. Our species has tamed the environment, and developed weapons of mass destruction, which make it easier to kill since we don't do it up close and personal. Our battles are fought over power, oil, ideology, and religion, none of which ensures survival of our species. Add to that mix the use of drugs, mild altering substances, and rational thought is adulterated, making it easier to kill. Thus, when we are left in total control we don't seem to do very well. Unlike other species, Homo sapiens *is* willing to kill other humans. We can certainly live without a spiritual connection, but we end up short-changed, without joy and serenity. Our egos are powerful forces, but when we assume total control, egos are capable of much misbehavior. The trick is to subordinate or align our egos to that of a higher power, God, and to live in the sunlight. We physicians can heal ourselves but we must want to heal ourselves.

The same is true of health care. Linear, reductionist methodology has become so imbedded in our lexicon that we are willing to apply whatever technology to a futile case, daring to challenge death, justifying our behavior with a commitment to the sanctity of life. We often carry out these ministrations distanced from our patients, hiding behind a microscope lens, sitting behind an x-ray machine, secure behind an endoscopic eye-piece or video screen, or insulated by anesthesia. We often misuse the fruits of science in malevolent ways, resulting in more misery for the dying patient, redefining life to suit high technology, allowing quality of life to be subordinated to "anything goes", and consuming valuable resources.

The challenge is to know when to use science, to understand and appreciate what it has to offer, yet to understand that we are not in complete control, that science is a gift from this loving and benevolent higher power, a gift that promises something better as we come to appreciate the fact that God's will does not hurt. Scientific endeavors, discoveries, inventions, and tools have a place in our lives, but left to our own devices, they can be harmful. With that in mind I believe that technomedicine can be harmful and this is much more likely to be the case as long as we technophysicians attempt to assume total control. As doctors, human beings, with the innate capacity to know right from wrong, we find ourselves in the cross-hairs of ill health ourselves when we indiscriminately succumb to inappropriate high technology. Like quality, the divine-human encounter becomes adulterated, subordinated, or just plain discarded by this cavalier attitude and, assuming complete control, we open the floodgates for spiritual bankruptcy and ill health. Many physicians today are struggling to stay in control, to find fulfillment, peace, prosperity, and longevity. They are working too hard, their hours are too long, they take chances, and they are more and more insensitive. Their goals have more to do with the bottom line than successfully ministering to their patients, an understandable fallout of spiritual bankruptcy. They are unhappy, petulant, and willing to blame anyone other than themselves. This is the portrait of a technophysician, the chief cause of the health care crisis. All of this has an impact on our patients who are placed at risk. I am once again reminded of the Evan's admonition that 95% of patients get well in spite of what we do. Fortunately, our patients survive in spite of ourselves, but that survival, without the all important process of becoming, leaves our patients at a disadvantage, without a spiritual connection, and barters away our opportunity for healing.

Today the votaries of technomedicine would probably label Dr. Fontaine, my professor from medical school, a relic of the past. They have abandoned the notion of the complete physician. They become so ensconced in their little niche of health care that they sacrifice the essential Marcus Welbian qualities of caring, communicating, feeling, and altruism. They are prepared to assault the patient with high technology and anything less is seen as a loss. They push for their particular technology regardless of the patient's misgivings, or preconceived notions. We technophysicians are patronizing, paternalistic, and dogmatic, seeing health care through our own very special lenses, without regard to less invasive alternatives. The very nature of high tech medicine invites supervening regulatory forces, primarily interested in cost control. Now, with their fingers now in the cookie jar, these dark side forces grapple with the technophysician for control, for a part of the doctor-patient action, making it easier for malevolent agencies to wrest away the physician's pen. We patients have stood by and let it happen! We have no one but ourselves to blame. But, it is not too late. We patients can still be involved.

We wounded healers, we technophysicians, now with incomplete, fragmented, and calcified egos, driven by nameless harpies, have become the single most important force in driving up health care expenditures. We have confused the sanctity of life with quality of life. Driven by the notion that life can always be resuscitated, resurrected, and repaired by technology, we come to believe that our preconceived notion of the sanctity of life is worth the effort. Dying and death are perfidious enemies, not worthy of our unbridled assault, not worthy of being part of the life process. Efforts to rescue elderly patients, enduring their natural death drama, although obscene, become the norm. Patients with futile conditions and terminal illness are routinely transferred to the intensive care units, where precious resources are consumed in a useless battle with Charon, who patiently awaits for that final trip across the River Styx. The last six months of life have become the most expensive for terminally ill Americans, who often become substrate for merciless, insensitive technophysicians, driven by faulty egos. Hospice has been a wonderful intervention in this situation, but it is often an afterthought. Soulful physicians have something to bring to the table here. Patient care conferences are the place where meaningful intervention is discussed, but one rarely sees technophysicians participating.

ICU nurses shake their heads, roll their eyes, and wonder amongst themselves what is the use of CPR for the elderly, cancer-ridden patient, whose ribs are broken by overzealous chest compression. It is not so much a notion of immortality, than the threat of personal failure, which drives technophyicians to implant internal pacemakers in patients with terminal cardiac disease. The nephrologist who initiates dialysis in the patient with multiple end organ failure, who is comatose, whose heart and lungs are failing, is dealing with a challenge to his expertise, or perhaps, a challenge to his concept of life and death. The gastroenterologist who attempts to remove a stone from the common bile duct of a demented patient with terminal pneumonia is more attuned to the technologic success of the procedure than the need for comfort with the inevitable dance of death. The ICU specialist who declines to remove any of the life support systems in the patient with a massive stroke has a perverted sense of success and a misunderstanding of death and dying.

It's not hard to see how technophysicians, swimming in a sea of discord, reach out for a convenient safe harbor, which is often greed, since emotional ballast is a best tenuous. We technophysicians substitute a financial riposte for emotional homeostasis. We have already discussed how this unsavory love affair has led to rising health care costs while imperiling health care at the same time. But this is no excuse. Technophysicians have taken advantage of a system that allows misbehavior, poor case selection, sloppy credentialing, inadequate self governance, and an educational system that looks the other way.

There is not a shred of evidence to support the notion that physicians are in some way spared the ravages of the human condition. The fall of man, original sin, or any of the ancient myths, which attempt to explain the foibles of mankind, is as applicable to physicians as to all of us. Thus, we physicians are skating on thin ice when we try to control everything, try to play God, ignoring for a moment the divine-human encounter. As a physician I learned this from Hank. We patients need to understand and accept this, demanding that physicians earn our faith, that we not be patronized, that we have an inherent right to be part of the healing process, to have a say, to play a meaningful role in decisions that are made. Physicians, particularly technphysicians, need to understand how to make themselves available for this line of inquiry. This skill needs to be taught and acquired in medical school and throughout the medical educational process. We need to be carefully educated by our physicians, physicians that we can trust, physicians who are willing and able to earn our trust. We need to accept and embrace those physicians whose answer to a question is "I don't know." We need to feel confident that they will find the correct answer. We patients need to know that physicians are simply human beings with special knowledge, but knowledge that might not be helpful if it is applied without soul. We need to understand that our health and well being are often subordinated to less savory motivations, that technophysicians often have a completely different mandate. In a life-threatening emergency we need to take a leap of faith, but not for most other situations.

The task is to repair Cartesian dualism. The separation of soma and psych has not furthered the cause of healing. Rather, it has led to the growth of technophysicians, who scandalously prostitute high technology for reasons that have more to do with their bottom line than our welfare. In the final chapters we will explore ways that the citizenry can make a difference, since this is the only group that has a chance of halting the inexorable downward course of our health care system. We are the ones who can demand more, thus reducing expenditures, without sacrificing quality, and ensure universal coverage without the need for big brother. Given the President's success in pushing through his version of health care reform, our task is to focus upon the protection of private health care, assuring that it becomes competitive with the public option, that quality is faithfully protected, and in so doing value is enhanced without cutting costs. Physicians must take this task seriously. They will need our encouragement and help. This is the message that I am trying to convey.

Chapter 16 Restoration: Cartesian Healing

I had always imagined a physician as some sort of magical person with a mysterious subliminal communication with his patient. When I was growing up, when I found myself in a doctor's office, my take of this person was that of an eminently wise, kindly, patient person, a gray haired man with a knowing smile, who could immediately connect with me and understand my problem. He (it was never a she when I was growing up) could assimilate all of the pieces of information that I gave him and make some sense out of it. There was an abiding faith on my part that he had my best interests at heart, that he would accept me, as I was, that I could be truthful without condemnation, and that my reward would be the restoration of my health. It was all so wonderful, this magical person with all of that knowledge, willing to dispense some to me so that I might get well. As a child it really never occurred to me that there was a fee, a price to be paid; there was nothing about his demeanor that led me to believe that I would be less worthwhile if money were not exchanged for services. Even as a child I was aware of what business transactions were. There was no room for small talk; there was no emotional or intuitive connection between the shop owner, only his willingness to give me what I had paid for. Not so with my doctor. Here there was an aura of confidence, a gift of knowledge, and a promise of healing. I was in the presence of a special person who cared enough about me to fix me, to take away the pain, to discharge me back into my world whole again.

I can still see my doctor' s eyes. They are soft, glistening, a little bloodshot, with baggy lids, a bit puffy, portals to accommodate all my rambling, my insecurities, my pain, and in essence they merged with me in a fundamental way that somehow led to my feeling better. O, there was always a stethoscope, lights to peer into my nose, ears and mouth, and hammers to test my reflexes. But, these instruments did not interpose a barrier between the two of us, did not stand in the way of this merger process, or of his intimate grasp of my condition. It was as if I were wrapped within some soft, warm garment, nourished, protected, and made to feel well. My concept of a doctor was someone who could envelop me with his caring, his wisdom, and provide me with a cocoon for my ultimate metamorphosis into health. Maybe it was akin to being in the womb, this warm and safe place where I first grew into wholeness. There was an unmistakable feminine texture to the process even though most of the doctors that I knew were men.

But that was in 1948 when I was eight years old. The avalanche of high technology was just beginning to make itself known, given its impetus from World War Two. Before long the business side of the equation would become much more important, replacing the gratuitous fabric of this intimate relationship with one much more impregnated with a monetary dimension. High technology would soon replace much of the intimate contact, which was commonplace between a doctor and patient. The promise of immortality, attested to by the victories over infectious diseases and battlefield injuries, were credentials for this new medicine and changed the essential nature of health care. This new paradigm, this exciting, glitzy, new world, offered seemingly impossible dreams, which were, in fact, impossible. But, that realization came later. The bifurcation between science and technology was launched. Given the dividends that technophysicians could expect, it did not take long for the momentum to pick up and invade the interstices of the health care industry.

Does the advent and progression of high technology necessarily eclipse the ideal of medicine, where an intimate relationship between physician and patient is created, much as what Dr. Fontaine and Mary Little established so many years ago? That is an essential question and at the heart of the matter. High technology was born of science and with that kind of pedigree it needs to be acknowledged. Yet, when it becomes the primary focus of health care, displacing or eclipsing other valid manners of healing, that becomes a problem. Can technophysicians embody the ideal? That is another important question. Given their focus on personal gain I think not. Technophysicians adulterate the honorable goals of this vocation. Thus, the task is to avoid the pernicious growth of technophysicians at the expense of this ideal. The goal is to treat the whole patient, and high technology is an important tool when applied appropriately.

Keep in mind that our health report card is at the bottom of the list compared to other industrialized nations. It is important to remember that in spite of spending nearly three trillion dollars on health care per year, nearly 16% of the gross domestic product, 40 million Americans are without health care insurance. Technophysicians are singularly responsible for driving the high technology engine and for driving up health care costs. We patients have let this happen and unless we cause change, the government will initiate draconian measures, which does not spell quality. National health may already be inevitable.

I am reminded of my first scientific conference. I was a trainee, a fellow in gastroenterology, and I was excited to attend this prestigious meeting. It was a baptism of sorts. Although not yet a bona fide gastroenterologist, I considered myself a member of this fraternity .New Orleans was a perfectly melded bouquet of Cajun, Creole, Black, Brown, White, Old South, French, Spanish, Antebellum and New South. The Mississippi River energized the city. The smells, sounds, tastes, and rhythm reached out and assaulted every one of my senses. Totally engulfed by this intoxicating blend, I felt so much a part of the moment. This was a different type of inebriation--one without a hangover, one that invaded all of my pores, one that healed and energized through assimilation.

Still, we were here to join medical researchers who were present to share their discoveries. We were all gathered to celebrate the advances of medical research, to learn new ways to probe the bodies of our patients, to measure and quantify disease, to offer new medicinal and surgical therapies for these perturbations, to claim victory over death and disease. It was heady stuff. The potent juices of New Orleans provided a healthy balm for our egos, insulating us against our own narcissism, offering a rhythmical counterpoint to excessive rationalism. I savored New Orleans while walking through the French Quarter, along Bourbon Street, by the Mississippi. The spontaneity and grace of the citizenry contrasted starkly with the demeanor of the visiting doctors. Once in the convention hall, there were thousands of physicians, mingling, deep in conversation, their serious studied faces occasionally breaking into fleeting smiles of recognition. They were all intent on learning, teaching, making a point, advancing with the tide of research. Their work was leading to new ways to treat ulcers, drugs to dissolve gallstones, drugs to suppress the activity of colitis, tools to stop gastric bleeding, to remove colonic polyps, and to relieve jaundice. All very heady stuff, a veritable smorgasbord of technology, a new repository of discovery, new facts, newly discovered enzymes, hormones, biochemical reactions, new markers of disease. Some of the best and brightest in medicine were there to cross-fertilize ideas, to share in discovery, to get a leg up on disease, to claim a new vantage of human illness, all confident that their work would be worthy. What a contrast! The city of New Orleans, steeped in history, the birthplace of jazz, swaying, swaggering, dipping to music that resonated with human vital forces, music that celebrated the totality of the human condition. This same city now invaded by top researchers and scientists whose work required that this same totality be invaded, probed, separated out, bits and pieces isolated, identified, described, and made ready for the successes of medical research.

After the plenary sessions, the convention got down to the work at hand. At any given moment there were ten separate scientific presentations going on, highlighting different aspects of the study of digestive disease and attended by small but still imposing audiences. The sessions were more or less divided by anatomy with meetings devoted to liver, gall bladder, colon, stomach, pancreas, esophagus, and so on.

I chose a meeting composed of physicians with an interest in ulcer diseases. It was one of the larger audiences, and nearly ten other scientific presentations preceded the one I remember most, the one which touched a nerve and made me think. Most of the presentations were by physicians from the U.S., Canada, the U.K., Australia and Israel. The demographics of the audience included fellows-in-training like myself, older and more seasoned researcher/teachers, private physicians, (primarily internists), gastroenterologists and surgeons. There were all types and shapes of attendees—guys with weird looking skull caps, little brown doctors from the third world with turbans, black guys sporting brightly colored shirts, professors in well worn suits, and a sprinkling of women, most of whom were curious wives.

The time had arrived. Almost as if in a dream, I heard the presenter's name announced, the title of his paper read, and suddenly he was walking toward the podium. He had worn a sports coat and slacks with a white shirt and paisley tie. Inside, the air conditioning was doing its job, but he was obviously drenched in sweat, his face flushed, his clothes sticking to his body. He stood at the podium, grabbed the edges with both hands, and tried to smile, or at least not look stupid. His presentation concerned itself with gastrin, a trophic hormone found in the stomach and measured in blood, which is very important in the genesis of peptic ulcer disease. A sea of eyes peered back at him. This was an amorphous mass of intellect, awaiting his first words, sitting quietly, expectantly, with mixed agendas. He began to talk. He stood at the podium, beads of sweat upon his brow, intent on reading from his notes, his eyes gazing up at intervals, furtively scanning the audience, steadying himself. Within an instant the amber light was on; it was time to wrap us his presentation. He seemed lost, not remembering what he had said, his mouth and brain on automatic pilot. He managed to approach the summary portion of his paper. By some quirk of fate, he peeled off his concluding sentence just before the red light. He had made it. Sweat poured down his face. His lips seemed parched and he seemed overwhelmed by thirst. He reached to pour himself a glass of water from the pitcher on the podium. He knocked both the pitcher and glass to the floor. Cold water coursed over his feet, tinkling with ice cubes. A busboy jumped to clean it up. There were a few perfunctory laughs from the audience and I blushed for him. The first questions were already coming.

Microphones were spaced throughout the auditorium for the benefit of those wishing to question the presenter. Some wanted to show off that they knew the literature better than him, that they had more sophisticated methodology, that they knew his mentors and felt the need to patronize him, but others had meaningful questions, curious about the techniques used, the clinical implications, the future direction of this research. In all, nearly ten persons asked questions, about the average, but it would have been much worse if no one had spoken up.

It was the last questioner that I vividly recall, who remains fixed in my mind, who left me unsettled, unsure, with more than just a modicum of discontent. He was an elderly white male, portly, in a sports coat like mine, with white hair combed back and horn-rimmed glasses. For a fleeting moment I thought he was my family physician. His face was kind but perplexed, somewhat confused. He cleared his throat. The room was very quiet. He congratulated the speaker on a well-organized presentation. I could see the presenter fill with pride. In a faint accent that I placed in the border-state region of the country-- Missouri or Indiana-- he asked how this line of research might benefit his ulcer patients. He was deadly serious, obviously intelligent, and spoke with a hint of sadness. I was confused. The other questioners had focused on the technical aspects of the paper, the methodology, and the interpretive piece. The dialogue was between scientific colleagues, a language born from the esoteric, built on the work of others. These questions were designed to help pave the way for the complete victory of science and technology in the larger arena of health care. Now here in front of me was the prototypical family physician, intellectually engaged, but with his obvious passion, his emotional dimension, listening and feeling for the presenter's response.

The presenter frowned. His eyes squinted, his forehead furrowed, he wrinkled his nose, and peered over the rim of his glasses. His answer was given deliberately, slowly, simmering in patronizing and pedantic juices. "Doctor, if you had been listening closely, you would recall that I said in my concluding remarks that by learning more about this hormone and its role in ulcer disease, new therapies would be forthcoming."

I have come to learn that the family physician was talking about outcomes, how much better off would his patient be, how much would suffering be reduced, not about curing an ulcer, not about healing a mucosal defect, not about whether surgery or medicine was more important. I have come to believe that he was talking about healing, a holistic re-righting of the disturbed organism, about the restoration the emotional, spiritual, and physical health of the affected person. He was not talking about what randomized clinical trials give us; about clinical outcomes or evidence-based medicine. He was talking about relevant bench to bedside issues, how he could be a better doctor utilizing relevant research, not delving into the methodological or statistical take of these matters.

The presenter carefully reminded this doctor about the path from the bench to the bedside. He carefully pointed out the future relevance of his paper. The doctor answered, "Thank you. I am sorry I may not have been listening as carefully as I might. I will reread your paper." There was a sprinkling of laughter amongst an otherwise very quiet audience. The amorphous mass of intellect shifted, coughed, and cleared its collective throat, betraying a moment of discomfort. I suddenly wanted to cry, to run into the arms of this caring physician, to apologize, but I was too proud, too much in love with myself, afflicted with unbridled narcissism, too caught up in this river of scientific endeavor, this intellectual feast, this preoccupation with soma.

And, so it is with technophysicians who are intent on blazing a path in the unknown and uncharted territory of future medical discoveries. A gulf develops which separates them from physicians intent on doing the best for their patients. It is not a calculated chasm, rather divergent paths that more often than not do not connect. We patients have persuaded our doctors to follow the path of the scientists, incorporating their findings into available diagnostic and therapeutic tools, making it easier for technophysicians to become surrogates for the scientists, making it easier for the inevitable separation of science from technomedicine. And ultimately, this drives up medical expenditures and puts our health care system into jeopardy.

Chapter 17
Into Action

The Sierra Nevada mountains tumble out of the Valley floor, rising gently to the east, born of the earth, molding and remolding, lingering in the wake of some long–lost glacier. A captivating view, a soothing balm to weary eyes, yet from this idyllic serenity one gets a sense of foreboding, as if the mountains might shrug should an unwary sojourner take these mammoths for granted. The gentle slopes of the Sierras have fooled more than one adventurer. The valley floor gives way to the trail head, rolling hills punctuated by the streams and rivers disgorging winter snows into the sea. In the spring the hills are an emerald green, wildflowers anoint the canyons, the blue sky is adorned by billowing white clouds, engaging all of the senses when one steps into this fairyland. The wise traveler gives this glacial monument its due, never assuming that nature's wilderness will let itself be tamed, staying respectful of creation, yet energized by its proximity.

The Sierras are a crucible where life's vicissitudes and human drama have played out: The tragedy of the Donner Party, the toil of the workers building the first transcontinental railroad, and the determination and loneliness of the Pony Express rider. These were all on my mind when several years removed from that day of graduation, on a beautiful early spring morning, with some fear and trepidation, I challenged these foothills with a bicycle ride.

My riding partner was Don Engle, an infectious–disease specialist, very outgoing, a seasoned mountain–bike rider, someone who could recharge his clinical acumen with forays into the gold country. Don was a bit older than me, but in a hell of a lot better shape. He rode a training bike every day to and from work, whatever the weather and his legs were beautifully contoured muscles that worked in tandem, meeting resistance with the power to shame the steepest slope. Don worked fantastically to stay in shape, peddling around town on an old beat–up three–speed, never skipping a day of riding to work.

The Sierra Nevadas were also a visual backdrop during my years in private practice. Snow capped in the winter, dark green and purple in the summer, they stood vigil over my growth and development as a physician. Gazing east, whether out of my office window, a hospital window, or through the windshield of my car, these mountains offered a border or boundary to all I could see and feel. They stood as a reminder of my own limitations, a sense of order during periods of chaos, and ballast for my own emotional and spiritual growth. But it was the bike ride with Don Engle that invited intimacy with these mountains and additional clarity into the cause of the health care crisis. My hip was healed, but running was out of the question and fortunately Don was not a runner.

I met Don early in practice. He seemed guarded, very careful, but willing to risk friendship. We had several patients in common and I had come to appreciate his clinical skills. He had a penchant for ferreting out useless information and reducing a febrile illness to the specific pathogenic microbe. He was supremely confident, seemingly without any imagination to conceive of failure, confidently perched atop the edifice of biomedicine, a little like Joseph Conrad's *Lord Jim*. An ode to Virchow, Koch, Pasteur, and Fleming, he could see nothing but virtue in the scientific method, that biomedical model that owed its existence to the 17th–century philosopher, Rene Descartes. Guys like Don made me comfortable with their notion that infectious scourges were on the way out, that scientific medicine had disease in full retreat. Ehrlich's magic bullet would lead us to Nirvana. It was just a matter of time. But, I still wondered.

A part time teacher at the medical school and highly respected in our community, Don was active in church and civic organizations. Quiet, attentive, lean, and balding, he had a peculiar nervous smile and a high pitched voice. He acted like he was mulling over what you had said, giving the impression of being respectful, but his mind was already made up, and it was unlikely that anything he saw, heard, or read would substantively change his opinion. Don must have thought I was a proficient bike rider. I had seen him once or twice on the river bike trail and I guess we had discussed bicycle equipment in the doctors lounge. In this instance I believe that he misjudged me. I was sure of it when he blurted out, "Hansen, let's do a fifty–miler."

We were munching bagels together in the doctors dining room when this gauntlet was thrown down. Though fairly certain that a fifty–miler was a bike ride amounting to fifty miles, I had no idea where the ride would take place. My riding had been limited to very flat surfaces, where there were lots of benches to sit upon and gaze at the river, where water fountains were plentiful, blessed with an abundance of shade trees, never far from home. I later learned that such amenities were anathema to Don. He disdained flat– landers, a pejorative for people who didn't venture into the foothills and mountains. Don impatiently waited for my answer, fidgeting, threatening to walk off before I had a chance to answer, leaving me to bathe in the juices of my uncertainty. So I sheepishly said, "Sure, why not."

So here we were, this agile and honed bicycle–riding machine and me. My bike was a 10 speed, like Don's, but without mountain gears. A disadvantage from the get– go. We had driven to a lake and unloaded our bikes. I could see where this road was headed from our point of disembarkation. It was going up, not flat, but up, and I didn't see any benches, shade trees, or water fountains. It was still early morning, with that something magical about the touch of a new born day. A sensuous freshness called out to all sense organs, to grasp the moment, to savor the delicious proximity. There were very few cars and the only noise I could hear other than my heart beating was the incessant melody of teeming insects. The lake was still, no wind yet, no white–caps, and on this Saturday morning newspapers had not yet been delivered. Beautiful homes dotted the lakeside but their owners were still asleep, comfortably snug in bed, not burdened with the uncertainty of a fifty–miler. God, what was I doing here?

I spent most of that day eating dust from Don's bike, frequently stopping for air, sweat pouring over my face, the muscles of my hands, legs, and arms burning, and wishing I was anywhere else. Don was reasonably patient and he tried to chat during those rest stops when I was gasping for air. An 8% grade doesn't sound like much. I reasoned that the other 92% must be flat-- a slight miscalculation. The way home was mostly downhill and we took it easy.

"Hansen, you're a lucky man to be a doctor."

I wasn't feeling terribly lucky at that moment, but I knew what he had in mind.

He went on to say, "The beauty of this profession is the precision available for burrowing to the root cause of sickness. The human body is so predictable. If you exercise regularly, it responds with more endurance and strength. If you abuse it, decay is inevitable."

Gasping for air, I related well to the decay part and managed to wheeze, "What about those cases where there doesn't appear to be an answer?"

He confidently answered, "In time science will give us the tools to answer every clinical question."

Well, that was that. There wasn't much else to say. Since the guy could ride so well, since he seemed able to walk the talk, I gave him the benefit of doubt. But is this all we want? Is this the kind of physician that infuses hope and soul into the equation? In one sense it doesn't matter how we answer this question because it is abundantly clear to me that Don's attitude fostered the overuse of high technology, a poor substitute for a spiritual connection, which contributes mightily to our health care crisis. We citizens deserve better and we must insist that we get better.

This is where spirituality comes in. I cannot foresee changes in our health care system until physicians are given the tools to achieve this. The universe offers more than clocklike precision, more than what Don was talking about. I believe that there is a higher power, one that may be different for each of us, one that is available to help each of us find answers, serenity, and peace. Without some connection to this celestial entity, all of us will be locked into the battle for control, which will inevitably and ultimately go against us if we are pitted against the universe. This is as true for physicians as or all of us. This process of connection is absolutely necessary if we are to create a new reality at the health care point of service. The techniques and skills needed to insure this connection for doctors would be left in the hands of physician educators, who understand and live this.

Spiritualism does not conflict with good science. As we unravel the secrets of the universe, our spiritual connection can and will grow if we are open minded. The restoration of meaningful health care, where soulful medicine and scientific medicine are joined, will facilitate the healing process. Ethical and moral considerations will become commonplace when physicians make decisions about the proper use of technology. Spirituality will provide the tools to move beyond the edges of science, where a situation appears to be futile and where hope has a place. Spirituality would provide physicians with answers and solutions to medical problems where there are no scientific answers. Spirituality creates a milieu where faith becomes a positive force, alleviating suffering and at the same time a source of strength for the physician. Spirituality provides a moral basis for decision-making; case selection is approached with honesty, diagnostic and therapeutic endeavors are brokered with veracity, instead of self serving motivation. Either directly or indirectly, physicians will include their patients as fellow travelers on the road towards spirituality. Much as Scott Peck wrote in *The Road Less Traveled*, physicians and their patients cash in on this spiritual journey, which replaces duplicity with honesty.

****

The Carnegie Institute is a privately funded, non-profit, organization created in 1902 and dedicated to the promotion of scientific discovery. In 1908 Abraham Flexner, a schoolmaster and educational theorist, was chosen by the Carnegie Institute at the behest of the AMA's Council of Medical Education, to investigate the process of medical education in the United States and to recommend a process of reform in an effort to achieve a single highest standard for those wishing to be doctors. This he did, instituting reforms, which inculcated the scientific method into the curricula, making medical education a very demanding endeavor. Thus, a layperson was able to singularly revolutionize medical education in America, paving the way for excellence in health care. This endeavor provided a standardized curricula, which has been a springboard from which allopathic medicine has sprung. It essentially insures that an individual who graduated from an American medical school and who has MD behind his name has been the recipient of a marvelous education.

At the time when Flexner embarked on this task most medical schools, or institutions that purported to educate new doctors, were proprietary. They were owned by the faculty, which often numbered no more than 7-8 persons. These physicians were part time teachers and the curricula was fragmented, often heavily weighted towards homeopathy. Flexner posited himself as the vanguard of philanthropy, an agent of the Carnegie Institute, which was commonly understood to be interested in funding these institutions. That gave Flexner a key to get in, to scrutinize these so-called teaching institutions , and unnoticed at the time, with an eye towards insuring that proper medical schools were adequately infused with scientific discovery. By raising the bar, his goal was to standardize the curricula. It was also to flush out substandard institutions, identifying those that were not including scientific information and scientific advancements in their programs. The result of his work was surprising for many of the schools that believed that he was simply there to arrange for philanthropic monies. The shock came when many of the substandard institutions were challenged to meet academic standards that were in fact impossible to meet. What Flexner did was to eliminate the for-profit schools, eliminating the need of the faculty to generate income, or run a for-profit shop, and thereby free the faculty from the tedious aspects of running a business. These teachers would no longer be encumbered with business matters and now able to focus on teaching. I don't believe that was his primary goal, but it was a byproduct of insisting that accredited medical schools inculcate medical advances into their curricula. Flexner did accomplish the goal of standardizing the curricula for medical schools, establishing an orthodoxy, demanding that all American medical schools adhere to the highest standards, and insuring the citizenry that anyone with an MD behind his name was the recipient of a robust education. What has actually happened during the past several years is the reverse of some of this process. Because medical schools have discovered the golden goose, having faculty perform procedures as a means of supporting a healthy revenue stream, teaching has dropped a notch, returning to a situation not unlike what Flexner had originally discovered. At the present time medical school faculty are up to their ears in generating income by doing procedures with less time to teach. Just think about it. A layperson, nearly by himself, revolutionized American medical education. The road map is clear. Citizens must become involved, much like Flexner, and lead us to the second medical educational revolution. In 1909 the establishment was reticent, much as it is today. But it can be done. This may be a way for the AMA to rejuvenate itself and take a leadership role in helping to find these teachers, who would develop a curriculum, which purports to make the study of spiritualism as it relates to health care a meaningful endeavor. This topic should be introduced to premedical students, continued throughout the four years of medical school, and throughout the postgraduate training, whatever that may be. It should be part of the continuing medical education process for practicing physicians who want to renew their licenses and board certification. Patients need to be satisfied that their doctors actively participate in this activity and certificates of attestation should be awarded.

This seed will take some time, but I am confident that health care will be well served. Infusing this new dimension should in no way turn back the clock of medical advancement, scientific discovery, and new technology. The point is to insure the appropriate use of new technology, which will pay dividends towards halting the escalating health care expenditures.

Can we do this again? We must or accept the consequences. There is a need to take inventory of the elements of spiritualism in the healing process, to assess how well these are included in medical education. These elements would include physicians use of prayer and meditation, reaching beyond themselves for faith based answers, understanding the value of a constant contact with our higher power, and the value that our higher power can do for us what we cannot do for ourselves. This would be a giant leap for the industry, but it something that needs to be done. This is not an inquisition, nor a religious exercise, nor a step back. This is an imperative and without commitment health care in America will suffer.

If the female side of the caduceus is resurrected, if the elements of spiritualism are made part of the healing process, then health care will be given a shot in the arm. The elements of allopathic medicine are in place, ready to be part of healing, but the task is help the medical-industrial complex awaken to this need. What I am proposing is a new Flexner Report, only this time rather than standardize the medical education curriculum, to rejuvenate this curriculum with the missing metaphysical piece, something that will enhance quality and infuse stewardship. Doctors don't need to be priests, rabbis or imams, rather invited to include the spiritual dimension along with modern medical technology, which will have a major impact on health care delivery in this country. This approach keeps physicians at the helm, obviating the need to include big brother.

Although Abraham Flexner did it by himself, I believe that it will take a motivated group of physicians to make it work today. It seems like such a far cry from what now is called medical education. But, we have to do something different. I believe that infusing spiritualism is the answer. This is no less than physicians availing themselves to the divine-human connection and availing themselves to the power, which derives from this celestial connection. This power will be available to physicians as they wrestle with judgment. This power will ensure the infusion of meaningful ethics into the day-to-day practice of medicine. This power will facilitate the proper application of altruism and empathy. Finally, this power will help physicians to minister to the whole person, to carefully listen to the patient, acknowledging that the patient is also part of this divine plan and is entitled to appropriate respect. But is this is just a dream? I think not.

Whatever we do, it will be the people driving this engine. Happily, we live in a democracy where our elected representatives are obliged to pay attention at the threat of losing their jobs. This is as it should be. First and foremost, however, it is incumbent upon us to become informed and to that extent I hope this book has been helpful. At the very least I hope this information becomes disseminated.

The heart of the American experience has been participatory democracy. When concerned individuals meet fact to face, their passion and will is fortified and the process will be lit up. This must happen if we are to be successful.

To be sure, there are things we can do in the meantime: Asking our physicians pertinent questions, demanding to be part of the order writing experience, understanding the difference between quality of life and sanctity of life, and paying attention to a healthy lifestyle. We must gather together, include physicians who understand what this is all about, and insist upon changes that have the potential to affect our health as well as the industry. In fact, as I have written, if the health care industry takes this seriously, premiums will drop, quality will rise, and this will obviate the need for government subsidized health care.

If we focus on these change, then it doesn't even require much involvement of our elected officials. If we are successful health care decisions will be left in the hands of physicians, but physicians who have learned that by including the spiritual dimension, ethical principles will lead to proper case selection, the proper use of high technology, good stewardship, and the return of the family doctor. This would certainly be a new approach, tilling new ground, and the process itself would require faith and hope, which are powerful forces to buttress change. The process would reorganize the practice of medicine to the extent that the spiritual dimension is included and at the same time not abandoning good science.

There is some debate about whether having too many specialists increases cost without necessarily improving quality. These studies have disparate results, bringing into question the methodology. CME or Medicare has been the major cash cow for graduate medical education. Several years ago CME capped the number of residencies that would be supported. The question is whether this number should be increased. I believe that a better goal is to insure that residents who participate in CME funded educational programs are properly educated with respect to the spiritual dimension, a path to soulful doctoring, the proper use of high technology, a meaningful approach to chronic disease, and the application of proper stewardship in areas such as the last six months of life and futile situations. This would be an appropriate use of federal funds. We must insist that this be done.

As citizens, we can ignore this call to arms, or discard the notion that there is an urgent need to repair the division that traces its origin to Descartes. But we do this at great peril. When we abandon holistic medicine we ask Big Brother to make health care decisions. These will be decisions made by lay persons, which will leave quality floundering. This is a poor substitute for health care reform. True health care reform is not a return to the Age of Faith, but one that down sizes humanism and includes spiritualism in health care decisions. This approach does not discount the marvelous scientific discoveries made during the past century; rather our science is given meaning. This celestial connection changes linear reductionism into holism.